Clean Eating Cookbook

125 Healthy Wholesome Recipes for Living a

Clean Eating Life

Aaron Mackellen

Table of Contents

Chapter 1: Breakfast Recipes..8

  Super-Healthy Juice (2 servings, serving: 1 glass) 8

  Green Goodness Juice (2 servings, serving: 1 glass) 9

  Berry Blast Smoothie (2 servings, serving: 1 glass)...10

  Tropical Smoothie (2 servings, serving: 1 glass)...11

  Fantastic Green Smoothie (2 servings, serving: 1 glass)..12

  Energizing Breakfast Bowl (3 servings, serving: 1 bowl) 13

  Berry Medley Bowl (3 servings, serving: 1 bowl)..14

  Busy Morning Breakfast (5 servings, serving: 1 portion)......................................15

  Nutrient Packed Granola (12 servings, serving: 1 portion) 16

  Wholesome Porridge (4 servings, serving: 1 portion) 18

  Healthier Porridge (6 servings, serving: 1 glass) 19

  Cold Morning Porridge (6 servings, serving: 1 portion) 20

  Satisfying Oatmeal (4 servings, serving: 1 portion) 21

  Overnight Oatmeal (3 servings, serving: 1 portion) 22

  Puffy Cherry Pancakes (4 servings, serving: 1 wedge) 23

  Pancakes (2 servings, serving: 1 pancake)...25

  Loveable Spicy Pancakes (6 servings, serving: 1 pancake).....................................27

  Deceptively Simple Waffles (2 servings, serving: 1 waffle)....................................29

  Crispy Waffles (4 servings, serving: 1 waffle)..30

  Extremely Yummy Muffins (5 servings, serving: 2 muffins) 31

  Extra-Special Muffins (12 servings, serving: 1 muffin) 32

  Versatile Tomato Muffins (12 servings, serving: 1 muffin).....................................34

  Thanksgiving Morning Bread (8 servings, serving: 1 slice) 36

  Fall-Time Breakfast Bread (14 servings, serving: 1 slice).......................................38

  Mediterranean Morning Bread (12 servings, serving: 1 slice)...............................40

  Super-Quick Omelet (4 servings, serving: 1 portion)..42

  Spanish Inspired Omelet (2 servings, serving: 1 portion)......................................44

  Effortless Scramble (2 servings, serving: 1 portion)...45

  Fluffy Scramble (7 servings, serving: 1 portion) 46

Best Vegan Scramble (2 servings, serving: 1 portion) 47

Favorite Quiche (3 servings, serving: 1 portion)..48

Green Garden Quiche (4 servings, serving: 1 portion) 49

Delish Breakfast Skillet (4 servings, serving: 1 portion) 51

Comforting Breakfast (2 servings, serving: 1 portion) 52

Nourishing Breakfast Hash (4 servings, serving: 1 portion)..................................54

Chapter 2: Lunch Recipes..56

Amazing Holiday Salad (5 servings, serving: 1 plate) 56

Tropical Salad (4 servings, serving: 1 plate)..58

Favorite Autumn Salad (8 servings, serving: 1 plate) 59

Warm Tofu Salad (4 servings, serving: 1 plate)..60

Vibrant Summer Salad (6 servings, serving: 1 plate) 62

Nutrient-Filled Soup (8 servings, serving: 1 bowl) 63

Garden Green Soup (4 servings, serving: 1 bowl) 64

Velvety Soup (5 servings, serving: 1 bowl)..65

Distinctive Veggie Soup (4 servings, serving: 1 bowl)..68

Aromatic Soup (6 servings, serving: 1 bowl) 70

Hearty Lettuce Wraps (4 servings, serving: 2 wraps) 72

Asian Style Lettuce Wraps (4 servings, serving: 2 wraps) 73

Flavor-Packed Burgers (4 servings, serving: 1 burger with 1 portion kale) 74

Awesome Burgers (8 servings, serving: 1 burger with 1 portion salad) 76

Foolproof Burgers (6 servings, serving: 1 burger with 1 portion arugula) 78

Classic Burgers (2 servings, serving: 1 burger with 1 portion salad) 80

Super-Tasty Meatballs (8 servings, serving: 1 portion meatballs & salad)..........82

Popular Winter Lunch (3 servings, serving: 1 portion) 84

Ideal Luncheon Meal (4 servings, serving: 1 portion) 85

Fuss-Free Lunch (2 servings, serving: 1 portion)..86

Healthy Veggie Combo (4 servings, serving: 1 portion) 87

Flavor-Packed Broccoli (2 servings, serving: 1 portion) 88

Glazed Carrots (4 servings, serving: 1 portion)..89

South-Asian Favorite Luncheon (4 servings, serving: 1 portion) 91

Garlicky Spinach (3 servings, serving: 1 portion)..93

Strengthening Meal (4 servings, serving: 1 portion)..95

Super-Food Luncheon (2 servings, serving: 1 portion)..96

Divine Veggie Pasta (4 servings, serving: 1 portion)..98

Super Healthy Lunch (4 servings, serving: 1 portion)..100

Refreshingly Tasty Meal (4 servings, serving: 1 portion)..101

Fabulous Tofu (2 servings, serving: 1 portion) 103

Irresistible Luncheon (3 servings, serving: 1 portion) 104

Naturally Nutritious Pilaf (3 servings, serving: 1 portion)......................................106

Amazingly Healthy Pilaf (4 servings, serving: 1 portion) 108

Colorful Salad (4 servings, serving: 1 plate)..109

Greek Style Salad (5 servings, serving: 1 plate)...110

All-in-One Salad (2 servings, serving: 1 plate)...111

Best-Ever Beef Salad (6 servings, serving: 1 plate)..113

Warming Soup (8 servings, serving: 1 bowl) 114

Beans Soup (8 servings, serving: 1 bowl) 116

Nutritive Soup (4 servings, serving: 1 bowl)..118

Popular Asian Soup (4 servings, serving: 1 bowl)...120

Thanksgiving Dinner Soup (8 servings, serving: 1 bowl) 122

Protein-Rich Stew (6 servings, serving: 1 bowl) 124

Creamy Chickpeas Stew (8 servings, serving: 1 bowl) 126

Scrumptious Stew (6 servings, serving: 1 bowl)...128

Great Entrée Stew (4 servings, serving: 1 bowl)...130

Omega-3 Rich Stew (6 servings, serving: 1 bowl) 132

Weeknight Dinner Chili (10 servings, serving: 1 bowl) 134

Richly Tasty Chili (8 servings, serving: 1 bowl)...136

Stunning Dinner Curry (4 servings, serving: 1 bowl)..138

Satisfying Curry (4 servings, serving: 1 bowl) 139

Lively Flavored Curry (4 servings, serving: 1 bowl)...141

Green Chicken Curry (5 servings, serving: 1 bowl)...143

Holiday Favorite Gratin (6 servings, serving: 1 portion)...145

Flavorsome Vegan Dinner (5 servings, serving: 1 portion) 147

Meat-Less Loaf (8 servings, serving: 1 portion) 150

Entertaining Casserole (6 servings, serving: 1 portion) 152

Decadent Casserole (5 servings, serving: 1 portion) 154

Party Dinner Casserole (3 servings, serving: 1 portion) 156

Enticing Casserole (6 servings, serving: 1 portion) 158

Flavorsome Chicken (4 servings, serving: 1 portion) 160

Deliciously Spicy Chicken (6 servings, serving: 1 portion) 162

Strengthening Dinner Meal (6 servings, serving: 1 portion) 164

Delish Chicken Platter (6 servings, serving: 1 portion) 166

Family Feast Dinner (5 servings, serving: 1 portion) 168

Succulent Lamb Chops (8 servings, serving: 1 portion) 169

Exceptionally Tasty Salmon (6 servings, serving: 1 portion) 171

Family Dinner Salmon (2 servings, serving: 1 portion) 172

Chapter 4: Snack Recipes 174

Appealing Party Treat (4 servings, serving: 1 portion) 174

Chunky Tomato Relish (3 servings, serving: 1 portion) 175

Naturally Sweet Guacamole (8 servings, serving: 1 portion) 176

Kids Friendly Fries (3 servings, serving: 1 portion) 177

Unique Pumpkin Seeds (6 servings, serving: 1 portion) 178

Welcoming Roasted Cashews (16 servings, serving: 1 portion) 179

Loveable Apple Leather (6 servings, serving: 1 portion) 180

Favorite Tea-Time Cookies (12 servings, serving: 1 portion) 181

Delectable Scones (7 servings, serving: 1 portion) 183

Fiesta Savory Treat (8 servings, serving: 1 portion) 185

Chapter 5: Dessert Recipes 187

Elegant Stuffed Apples (4 servings, serving: 1 apple) 187

Summery Mango Delight (6 servings, serving: 1 portion) 189

Creamy Ice-Cream (6 servings, serving: 1 portion) 190

Refreshing Granita (8 servings, serving: 1 portion) 192

Classic Pudding (3 servings, serving: 1 portion) 193

Family Favorite Pudding (4 servings, serving: 1 portion) 194

Traditional Holiday Pudding (4 servings, serving: 1 portion) 195

Sweet-Tooth Carving Custard (8 servings, serving: 1 portion) 196

Thanksgiving Party Mousse (4 servings, serving: 1 portion) 197

Luscious Cheesecake (8 servings, serving: 1 portion) 199

Stunning Strawberry Sundae (2 servings, serving: 1 portion) 200

Celebratory Crisp (8 servings, serving: 1 portion) 201

Exotic Crumble (4 servings, serving: 1 portion)..203

Kid's Favorite Mini Cakes (6 servings, serving: 1 mini cake)..204

Quickest Zesty Cake (1 serving, serving: 1 cake) 206

CHAPTER 1: BREAKFAST RECIPES

Super-Healthy Juice (2 servings, serving: 1 glass)

Per Serving, Calories: 228- Fat: 0.8g - Carbs: 58.7g - Protein: 2.5g

Ingredients:

- 3 cored and sliced large Granny Smith apples

- 3 peeled and chopped medium carrots

- 1 sliced large tomato

Directions:

1. In a juicer, add all ingredients and extract the juice according to manufacturer's directions.

2. Transfer into 2 glasses and serve immediately.

Green Goodness Juice (2 servings, serving: 1 glass)

Per Serving, Calories: 366- Fat: 1.3g - Carbs: 90.2g - Protein: 6.3g

Ingredients:

- 4 large peeled, seeded and sectioned oranges

- 3 cored and sliced medium green apples

- 2 chopped broccoli stalks

- ¼ cup of fresh parsley leaves

Directions:

1. In a juicer, add all ingredients and extract the juice according to manufacturer's directions.

2. Transfer into 2 glasses and serve immediately.

Berry Blast Smoothie (2 servings, serving: 1 glass)

Per Serving, Calories: 79- Fat: 0.5g - Carbs: 18.7g - Protein: 2.1g

Ingredients:

- 1 cup of frozen strawberries

- ½ cup of frozen blueberries

- ½ cup of frozen blackberries

- ¼ cup of frozen cranberries

- 3 cups of fresh spinach

- ½ tsp. of peeled and chopped fresh ginger

- 1 cup of filtered water

Directions:

1. In a high speed blender, add all ingredients and pulse till smooth.
2. Transfer into 2 glasses and serve immediately.

Tropical Smoothie (2 servings, serving: 1 glass)

Per Serving, Calories: 135- Fat: 3.2g - Carbs: 28.7g - Protein: 1.8g

Ingredients:

- 1 cup of chopped frozen pineapple

- 1 cup of peeled, pitted and chopped frozen mango

- 1 cup of peeled and chopped papaya

- 1 tsp. of ground turmeric

- ½ tsp. of ground ginger

- ½ tsp. of ground cinnamon

- 1½ cups of unsweetened almond milk

Directions:

1. In a high speed blender, add all ingredients and pulse till smooth.
2. Transfer into 2 glasses and serve immediately.

Fantastic Green Smoothie (2 servings, serving: 1 glass)

Per Serving, Calories: 174- Fat: 1.8g - Carbs: 40.6g - Protein: 1.3g

Ingredients:

- 2 cups of trimmed collard greens

- 2 cups of seedless green grapes

- 1 tbsp. of maple syrup

- 1½ cups of filtered water

- ¼ cup of ice cubes

Directions:

1. In a high speed blender, add all ingredients and pulse till smooth.
2. Transfer into 2 glasses and serve immediately.

Energizing Breakfast Bowl (3 servings, serving: 1 bowl)

Per Serving, Calories: 194- Fat: 3.8g - Carbs: 42g - Protein: 4.1g

Ingredients:

- 2 cups of pitted frozen cherries

- 4 pitted and chopped dates

- 1 peeled, cored and chopped large apple

- 1 cup of fresh cherries, pitted

- 2 tbsp. of chia seeds

Directions:

1. In a high speed blender, add frozen cherries and dates and pulse till smooth.

2. In a large bowl, mix together apple, fresh cherries and chia seeds.

3. Add cherry sauce and stir to combine.

4. Cover and refrigerate to chill for overnight.

Berry Medley Bowl (3 servings, serving: 1 bowl)

Per Serving, Calories: 189- Fat: 4g - Carbs: 22.5g - Protein: 18.6g

Ingredients:

- 2 cups of fat-free plain Greek yogurt

- 1 cup of fresh blueberries

- 1 cup of fresh blackberries

- 1 cup of hulled and sliced fresh strawberries

- 2 tbsp. of chopped walnuts

Directions:

1. In a large bowl, add yogurt.

2. Add remaining ingredients and gently, stir to combine.

3. Divide into 2 serving bowls and serve immediately.

Busy Morning Breakfast (5 servings, serving: 1 portion)

Per Serving, Calories: 346- Fat: 8.6g - Carbs: 67.1g - Protein: 7.1g

Ingredients:

- 1¾ cups of unsweetened almond milk

- 6 pitted and chopped Medjool dates

- 1 tbsp. of organic vanilla extract

- 2 (10-ounce) packages of thawed frozen raspberries

- ½ cup of chia seeds

Directions:

1. In a food processor, add all ingredients except chia seeds and pulse till smooth.

2. Transfer the mixture in a large bowl.

3. Add chia seeds and stir to combine well.

4. Refrigerate for about 4-6 hours, stirring occasionally.

Nutrient Packed Granola (12 servings, serving: 1 portion)

Per Serving, Calories: 295- Fat: 14.5g - Carbs: 39.3g - Protein: 7.6g

Ingredients:

- 2 cups of oats

- 1 cup of buckwheat groats

- 1 cup of pumpkin seeds

- 1 cup of sunflower seeds

- 1½ cups of pitted and chopped fresh dates

- 1 cup of fresh apple puree

- 1/3 cup of extra-virgin olive oil

- 1 tsp. of finely grated fresh ginger

- ¼ cup of raw cacao powder

Directions:

1. Preheat the oven to 355 degrees F. Grease a large baking dish.

2. In a large bowl, add oats, buckwheat and seeds and mix well.

3. In a pan, mix together dates, apple puree and oil on medium-low heat and simmer for about 5 minutes, stirring continuously.

4. Stir in ginger and immediately remove from heat.

5. Keep aside to cool slightly.

6. In a blender, add date mixture and cacao powder and pulse till a smooth mixture forms.

7. Add the date mixture in the bowl with oat mixture and stir to combine well.

8. Transfer the mixture into prepared baking dish evenly.

9. Bake for about 15 minutes.

10. Remove from oven and stir well.

11. Bake for about 30 minutes, stirring after every 5-10 minutes.

12. This granola can be preserved in an airtight container.

Wholesome Porridge (4 servings, serving: 1 portion)

Per Serving, Calories: 137- Fat: 4.7g - Carbs: 24.6g - Protein: 2.2g

Ingredients:

- 2 cups of unsweetened almond milk
- 2 peeled, cored and grated large apples
- 3 tbsp. of sunflower seeds
- ¼ tsp. of ground cinnamon
- ½ tsp. of organic vanilla extract
- ½ cup of fresh blueberries
- ½ cup of peeled and sliced banana
- 2 tbsp. of toasted and chopped almonds

Directions:

a. In a large pan, mix together almond milk, apples, sunflower seeds, cinnamon and vanilla extract on medium-low heat.

b. Cook gently, stirring occasionally for about 3-4 minutes.

c. Remove from heat and transfer into serving bowls. Let it cool slightly.

d. Top with blueberries and banana slices evenly.

e. Garnish with almonds and serve.

Healthier Porridge (6 servings, serving: 1 glass)

Per Serving, Calories: 94- Fat: 3.5g - Carbs: 16.4g - Protein: 1.1g

Ingredients:

- ½ cup of grated into rice like consistency cauliflower

- 2 cups of peeled, cored and shredded apple

- ½ cup of shredded unsweetened coconut

- 1¾ cups of unsweetened almond milk

- 1 tsp. of organic vanilla extract

- ½ cup of peeled and sliced banana

- 1/3 cup of fresh blueberries

Directions:

1. In a large pan, mix together all ingredients except blueberries on medium heat and bring to a gentle simmer.
2. Reduce the heat to low and simmer for about 15-20 minutes, stirring occasionally.
3. Serve warm with the topping of blueberries.

Cold Morning Porridge (6 servings, serving: 1 portion)

Per Serving, Calories: 282- Fat: 11.2g - Carbs: 39.1g - Protein: 8.1g

Ingredients:

- 3½ cups of filtered water

- 1¾ cups of soaked for 15 minutes and rinsed quinoa

- 14-ounce of unsweetened almond milk

- 1¾ cups of homemade pumpkin puree

- 2 tsp. of ground cinnamon

- 1 tsp. of ground ginger

- Pinch of sea salt

- 3 tbsp. of olive oil

- 6-8 drops of liquid stevia

- 1 tsp. of organic vanilla extract

Directions:

1. In a pan, add water and quinoa on high heat.

2. Cover and bring to a boil.

3. Reduce the heat to low and simmer for about 12 minutes or till all the liquid is absorbed.

4. Add remaining ingredients and stir till well combined.

5. Serve warm.

Satisfying Oatmeal (4 servings, serving: 1 portion)

Per Serving, Calories: 163- Fat: 3.1g - Carbs: 31.8g - Protein: 3.2g

Ingredients:

- 2 cups of unsweetened almond milk

- 1¼ cups of filtered water

- 2 tbsp. of honey

- 1 peeled, cored and chopped apple

- ¼ cup of fresh cranberries

- 2 cups of old-fashioned oats

- ½ tsp. of ground cinnamon

- 1 tsp. of organic vanilla extract

Directions:

1. In a pan, add almond milk, water, honey, apple and cranberries on medium heat and bring to a boil.

2. Add oats and cinnamon and cook for about 3-5 minutes, stirring occasionally.

3. Stir in vanilla and remove from the heat.

4. Serve warm.

Overnight Oatmeal (3 servings, serving: 1 portion)

Per Serving, Calories: 360- Fat: 9g - Carbs: 64.3g - Protein: 9.3g

Ingredients:

For Sweet Potato:

- 2 cups of cooked, peeled and chopped sweet potato

- 1 cup of unsweetened almond milk

- ½ tsp. of ground cinnamon

For Oatmeal:

- 1 cup of rolled oats

- 1 cup of unsweetened almond milk

- 2 tbsp. of chia seeds

- 2 tbsp. of honey

- ½ tsp. of organic vanilla extract

- 1 tbsp. of chopped pecans

Directions:

1. For sweet potato puree in a blender, add all ingredients and pulse till smooth.

2. Transfer the mixture into a bowl and refrigerate, covered for overnight.

3. In another medium bowl, add all oatmeal ingredients except pecans and mix until well combined.

4. Refrigerate, covered for overnight.

5. In the morning, remove from the refrigerator.

6. Layer the oatmeal and sweet potato puree in a serving bowls evenly.

7. Top with pecans and serve.

Puffy Cherry Pancakes (4 servings, serving: 1 wedge)

Per Serving, Calories: 209- Fat: 11.5g - Carbs: 19.4g - Protein: 7.7g

Ingredients:

- 1 tbsp. plus 1 tsp. of olive oil, divided

- ½ cup of gluten-free whole-wheat flour

- 1/8 tsp. of ground cinnamon

- Pinch of sea salt

- 3 organic eggs

- ½ cup of unsweetened almond milk

- 1 tsp. of organic vanilla extract

- 2 cups of pitted and halved fresh sweet cherries

- ¼ cup of chopped almonds

Directions:

1. Preheat the oven to 450 degrees F.

2. In a 10-inch ovenproof skillet, add 1 tsp. of oil and place the skillet into oven.

3. In a bowl, mix together flour, cinnamon and salt.

4. In another bowl, add eggs, almond milk, remaining oil and vanilla extract and beat till well combined.

5. Add egg mixture into flour mixture and mix till well combined.

6. Remove the skillet from oven and tilt to spread the oil evenly.

7. Place cherries in the bottom of skillet in a single layer.

8. Place the flour mixture over cherries evenly and top with almonds evenly.

9. Bake for about 15-20 minutes or till a toothpick inserted in the center comes out clean.

10. Remove from oven and let it cool for at least 5 minutes before slicing.

11. Cut into 4 equal sized wedges and serve.

Pancakes (2 servings, serving: 1 pancake)

Per Serving, Calories: 197- Fat: 10.3g - Carbs: 19.9g - Protein: 9.5g

Ingredients:

- ¼ cup of arrowroot flour

- ¼ cup rolled oats

- ¼ tsp. of baking soda

- ½ tsp. of baking powder

- 1/8 tsp. of ground cinnamon

- ¼ cup of unsweetened almond milk

- 2 organic egg whites

- 2 tsp. of almond butter, divided

- ½ of peeled and mashed banana

- 1/8 tsp. of organic vanilla extract

Directions:

1. In a large bowl, mix together oats, flour, baking soda, baking powder and cinnamon.

2. In another bowl, add milk, egg whites, 1 tsp. of almond butter, banana and vanilla and beat till well combined.

3. Add flour mixture into milk mixture and mix till well combined.

4. Grease a large frying pan with remaining butter on low heat.

5. Add half of mixture and cook for about 1-2 minutes per side.

6. Repeat with the remaining mixture.

Loveable Spicy Pancakes (6 servings, serving: 1 pancake)

Per Serving, Calories: 219- Fat: 15.5g - Carbs: 21.3g - Protein: 1.6g

Ingredients:

- ½ cup of almond flour

- ½ cup of tapioca flour

- ½ tsp. of chili powder

- ¼ tsp. of ground turmeric

- Sea salt and freshly ground black pepper, to taste

- 1 cup of unsweetened coconut milk

- ½ of chopped red onion

- ¼ tsp. of finely grated fresh ginger

- 1 seeded and minced Serrano pepper

- ½ cup of chopped fresh cilantro

- 2 tbsp. of canola oil

Directions:

1. In a large bowl, mix together flours and spices.

2. Add coconut milk and mix till well combined.

3. Fold in the onion, ginger, Serrano pepper and cilantro.

4. Lightly, grease a large nonstick skillet with oil and heat on medium-low heat.

5. Add about ¼ cup of mixture and tilt the pan to spread it evenly in the skillet.

6. Cook for about 3-4 minutes from both sides.

7. Repeat with the remaining mixture.

Deceptively Simple Waffles (2 servings, serving: 1 waffle)

Per Serving, Calories: 99- Fat: 0.9g - Carbs: 11.8g - Protein: 11.2g

Ingredients:

- ¼ cup of coconut flour

- 1 tsp. of baking powder

- ¼ cup of unsweetened almond milk

- 6 organic egg whites

- 1 tbsp. of honey

- Dash of organic vanilla extract

Directions:

1. Preheat the waffle iron and lightly grease it.

2. In a large bowl, add flour and baking powder and mix well.

3. Add remaining ingredients and mix till well combined.

4. Place half of the mixture in preheated waffle iron.

5. Cook for about 3-4 minutes or till waffles become golden brown.

6. Repeat with the remaining mixture.

7. Serve warm.

Crispy Waffles (4 servings, serving: 1 waffle)

Per Serving, Calories: 71- Fat: 0.3g - Carbs: 16.2g - Protein: 1.6g

Ingredients:

- 2 peeled, grated and squeezed medium sweet potatoes

- 1 tbsp. of minced chives

- 1 tbsp. of minced fresh rosemary

- ¼ tsp. of crushed red pepper flakes

- Sea salt and freshly ground black pepper, to taste

Directions:

1. Preheat the waffle iron and then grease with cooking spray.

2. In a large bowl, add all ingredients and mix till well combined.

3. Place ¼ of the sweet potato mixture into preheated waffle iron.

4. Cook for 8-10 minutes or till golden brown.

5. Repeat with the remaining mixture.

Extremely Yummy Muffins (5 servings, serving: 2 muffins)

Per Serving, Calories: 78- Fat: 3.5g - Carbs: 8.6g - Protein: 3.3g

Ingredients:

- ½ cup of rolled oats

- ¼ cup almond flour

- 2 tbsp. of flaxseeds

- ½ tsp. of baking soda

- ½ tsp. of ground cinnamon

- 1 organic egg

- ¼ cup of almond butter

- 2 tbsp. of mashed banana

- ¼ cup of fresh blackberries

Directions:

1. Preheat the oven to 375 degrees F. Grease 10 cups of a muffin tin.

2. In a blender, add all ingredients except blackberries and pulse till smooth and creamy.

3. Transfer the mixture into a bowl and fold in the blackberries.

4. Transfer the mixture into prepared muffin cups evenly.

5. Bake for about 10-12 minutes or till a toothpick inserted in the center comes out clean.

Extra-Special Muffins (12 servings, serving: 1 muffin)

Per Serving, Calories: 196- Fat: 10.2g - Carbs: 24.4g - Protein: 5.3g

Ingredients:

- 2 cups of blanched almond meal

- ½ cup of unsweetened coconut shreds

- 1 tsp. of baking soda

- ½ tsp. of ground allspice

- Pinch of ground cardamom

- Pinch of sea salt

- 3 organic eggs

- ½ cup of honey

- ½ cup of canola oil

- 1 cup of peeled and grated carrot

- 2 tbsp. of peeled and grated fresh ginger

- ¾ cup of soaked in water for 15 minutes and drained raisins

Directions:

1. Preheat the oven to 350 degrees F. Grease 12 cups of a large muffin tin.

2. In a large bowl, add flour, coconut shreds, baking soda, spices and salt and mix well.

3. In another bowl, add the eggs, honey, and oil and beat till well combined.

4. Add egg mixture into flour mixture and mix till well combined.

5. Gently, fold in carrot, ginger and raisins.

6. Place the mixture into prepared muffin cups evenly.

7. Bake for about 20-22 minutes or till a toothpick inserted in the center comes out clean.

8. Remove the muffin tin from oven and keep on wire rack to cool for about 10 minutes.

9. Carefully turn on a wire rack to cool completely before serving.

Versatile Tomato Muffins (12 servings, serving: 1 muffin)

Per Serving, Calories: 94- Fat: 6.8g - Carbs: 2.6g - Protein: 6.1g

Ingredients:

- 12 organic eggs

- ½ cup of unsweetened coconut milk

- 1 tsp. of ground turmeric

- Sea salt and freshly ground black pepper, to taste

- 1 cup of chopped tomatoes

- 1 cup of chopped spinach

- ½ cup of seeded and chopped green bell peppers

- ½ cup of chopped onions

- 1 minced garlic clove

- 1 tbsp. of chopped fresh basil

Directions:

1. Preheat the oven to 350 degrees F. Grease 12 cups of a large muffin tin.

2. In a large bowl, add eggs, coconut milk, turmeric, salt and black pepper and neat till well combined.

3. Add remaining ingredients and mix till well

4. Place the mixture into prepared muffin cups evenly.

5. Bake for about 15 minutes or till a toothpick inserted in the center comes out clean.

6. Remove the muffin tin from oven and keep on wire rack to cool for about 10 minutes.

7. Carefully turn on a wire rack and serve warm.

Thanksgiving Morning Bread (8 servings, serving: 1 slice)

Per Serving, Calories: 214- Fat: 14.6g - Carbs: 16.1g - Protein: 5.9g

Ingredients:

- 2/5 cup of coconut flour

- ½ tsp. of baking soda

- ½ tsp. of baking powder

- ¼ tsp. of ground cinnamon

- ¼ tsp. of ground cardamom

- Pinch of sea salt

- 6 large organic eggs

- 1/3 cup of honey

- 1/3 cup of extra-virgin olive oil

- ½ cup of fresh orange juice

- ½ tbsp. of organic vanilla extract

- 1 cup of fresh cranberries

- ¼ cup of chopped walnuts

- 1 tbsp. of finely grated fresh orange zest

Directions:

1. Preheat the oven to 350 degrees F. Line a loaf pan with parchment paper.

2. In a large bowl, mix together flour, baking soda, baking powder, spices and salt.

3. In another bowl, add eggs, honey, oil, orange juice and vanilla extract and beat till well combined.

4. Add egg mixture into flour mixture and mix till just combined.

5. Fold in cranberries, walnuts and orange zest.

6. Transfer the mixture into prepared loaf pan evenly.

7. Bake for about 45-50 minutes or till a toothpick nested in the center comes out clean.

8. Remove the bread pan from oven and keep on wire rack to cool for about 5 minutes.

9. Carefully turn on a wire rack and to cool completely before serving.

10. Cut into desired slices and serve.

Fall-Time Breakfast Bread (14 servings, serving: 1 slice)

Per Serving, Calories: 151- Fat: 5.6g - Carbs: 23.6g - Protein: 2.6g

Ingredients:

- 1¾ cups of gluten-free whole wheat flour

- ½ tsp. of ground cinnamon

- ½ tsp. of ground ginger

- ¼ tsp. of ground nutmeg

- 1/8 tsp. of ground cardamom

- 1/8 tsp. of ground cloves

- Sea salt, to taste

- 2 organic eggs

- ½ cup of honey

- 1/3 cup of extra-virgin olive oil

- 1 cup of homemade pumpkin puree

- 1 tsp. of organic vanilla extract

- 1 tsp. of baking soda

- ¼ cup of hot water

Directions:

1. Preheat the oven to 325 degrees F. Grease a 9x5-inch loaf pan.

2. In a bowl, mix together flour, spices and salt.

3. In another large bowl, add eggs, honey and oil and beat till well combined.

4. Add flour mixture and mix till just combined.

5. In a bowl, dissolve the baking soda in hot water.

6. Slowly, add baking soda mixture into flour mixture and mix till well combined.

7. Transfer the mixture into prepared loaf pan evenly.

8. Bake for about 55-65 minutes or till a toothpick inserted in the center comes out clean.

9. Remove bread from oven and let it cool slightly before slicing.

10. Remove the bread pan from oven and keep on wire rack to cool for about 5 minutes.

11. Carefully turn on a wire rack and to cool completely before serving.

12. Cut into desired slices and serve.

Mediterranean Morning Bread (12 servings, serving: 1 slice)

Per Serving, Calories: 200- Fat: 6.6g - Carbs: 29.7g - Protein: 6.1g

Ingredients:

- ½ cup of pitted and chopped black olives

- ¼ cup of fresh thyme

- 2 tbsp. of extra-virgin olive oil

- 4 pitted dates

- ½ cup of hemp seeds

- 1½ cups of filtered water

- 3 cups of whole wheat flour

- ¼ cup of chia seeds

- 4 tsp. of baking powder

- 1/8 tsp. of crushed red pepper flakes

- Sea salt and freshly ground black pepper, to taste

Directions:

1. Preheat the oven to 400 degrees F. Arrange the rack in the bottom third of oven.
2. Lightly, grease a bread loaf pan.

3. In a food processor, add olives, thyme and oil and pulse till well combined.

4. Transfer the olive mixture into a bowl.

5. In a high speed blender, add dates, hemp seeds and water and pulse till well combined.

6. Transfer the date mixture into another bowl.

7. In a large bowl, mix together flour, chia seeds, baking powder, red pepper flakes, salt and black pepper.

8. Add olives mixture into flour mixture and mix till just moistened.

9. Make a well in the flour mixture.

10. Add the date mixture in the well and with a fork gently, mix till well combined.

11. Place the dough onto a lightly floured surface.

12. With lightly floured hands, knead the dough and form into an oblong loaf.

13. Transfer the loaf into prepared loaf pan, seam side down.

14. With a knife, make 2 (½-inch) deep diagonal cuts in the center of loaf.

15. Dust the loaf with a little flour.

16. With a kitchen towel, cover the pan and keep aside for about 10 minutes.

17. Bake for about 50-55 minutes or till top becomes golden brown.

18. Remove the bread pan from oven and keep on wire rack to cool for about 10-15 minutes.

19. Carefully turn on a wire rack and serve warm.

Super-Quick Omelet (4 servings, serving: 1 portion)

Per Serving, Calories: 164- Fat: 7.4g - Carbs: 3.3g - Protein: 20.4g

Ingredients:

- 1 cup of halved grape tomatoes

- 2 tbsp. of extra-virgin olive oil, divided

- 1 tbsp. of fresh lemon juice

- Sea salt and freshly ground black pepper, to taste

- 3 cups of organic egg whites

- ½ cup of chopped fresh cilantro leaves

Directions:

1. Preheat the broiler to high heat. Set an oven rack near the broiler.

2. In a large bowl, add tomatoes, 1 tsp. of oil, lemon juice, a pinch of salt and black pepper and toss to coat well.

3. Cover and keep aside for at least 10-15 minutes.

4. In a large bowl, add egg whites, cilantro, a little salt and black pepper and beat till foamy.

5. In an ovenproof skillet heat the remaining oil on medium-low heat.

6. Add the egg whites mixture and swirl to cover the whole skillet.

7. Cook, without stirring for about 3-4 minutes or till the whites are almost set.

8. Place half of marinated tomatoes over half portion of the omelet.

9. Carefully fold the omelet over the tomatoes.

10. Immediately, transfer the skillet under the broiler and broil for about 1 minute.

11. Divide the omelet into serving plates and serve with the topping of remaining tomatoes.

Spanish Inspired Omelet (2 servings, serving: 1 portion)

Per Serving, Calories: 192- Fat: 13.8g - Carbs: 2.6g - Protein: 14.9g

Ingredients:

- 4 large organic eggs

- 2 tbsp. of chopped onion

- 2 tbsp. of chopped fresh parsley

- Pinch of sea salt

- 1 tsp. of extra-virgin olive oil

- ¼ cup of cooked and squeezed spinach

- 1-ounce of crumbled low-fat goat cheese

Directions:

1. In a bowl, add the eggs, onion, parsley, salt and black pepper and beat well.

2. In a nonstick frying pan, heat oil on medium heat.

3. Add egg mixture and tilt the skillet to spread the mixture evenly.

4. Cook for about 3minutes or till set completely.

5. Place spinach and feta over the omelet and carefully lift one side to fold the omelet.

6. Reduce the heat to medium-low and cook for about 1 minute.

Effortless Scramble (2 servings, serving: 1 portion)

Per Serving, Calories: 225- Fat: 15.9g - Carbs: 8.8g - Protein: 13.2g

Ingredients:

- 4 organic eggs

- 1 tbsp. of olive oil

- 2 cups of trimmed and chopped fresh kale

- 1½ tsp. of ground turmeric

- Sea salt and freshly ground black pepper, to taste

Directions:

1. In a bowl, add eggs and beat well.

2. In a nonstick skillet, heat oil on medium heat.

3. Add kale and cook for about 2 minutes.

4. Add eggs and remaining ingredients cook for about 3-4 minutes or till desired doneness, stirring continuously.

Fluffy Scramble (7 servings, serving: 1 portion)

Per Serving, Calories: 188- Fat: 14.3g - Carbs: 2.4g - Protein: 3.3g

Ingredients:

- 2 tbsp. of olive oil

- 1 chopped jalapeño pepper

- 1 chopped small red onion

- 12 lightly beaten large organic eggs

- Sea salt and freshly ground black pepper, to taste

- 3 tbsp. of finely chopped chives

- 4-ounce of crumbled low-fat goat cheese

Directions:

1. In a large skillet, heat oil on medium heat.

2. Add jalapeño pepper and onion and sauté for about 4-5 minutes.

3. Add eggs, salt and black pepper and cook for about 3 minutes, stirring continuously.

4. Remove from heat and immediately, stir in chives and cheese.

5. Serve immediately.

Best Vegan Scramble (2 servings, serving: 1 portion)

Per Serving, Calories: 213- Fat: 11.8g - Carbs: 14.7g - Protein: 17.3g

Ingredients:

- ½ tbsp. of extra-virgin olive oil

- 1 finely chopped small onion

- 1 seeded and finely chopped small red bell pepper

- 1 cup of finely chopped cherry tomatoes

- 1½ cups of pressed and crumbled firm tofu

- Pinch of ground turmeric

- Pinch of cayenne pepper

- 1 tbsp. of chopped fresh parsley

Directions:

1. In a skillet, heat oil on medium heat.

2. Add onion and bell pepper and sauté for about 4-5 minute.

3. Add tomatoes and cook for about 1-2 minutes.

4. Add tofu, turmeric and cayenne pepper and cook for about 6-8 minutes, stirring continuously.

5. Garnish with parsley and serve.

Favorite Quiche (3 servings, serving: 1 portion)

Per Serving, Calories: 120- Fat: 7.4g - Carbs: 3.9g - Protein: 9.9g

Ingredients:

- 5 organic eggs

- Sea salt and freshly ground black pepper, to taste

- 1 peeled and grated carrot

- 1 shredded small zucchini

Directions:

1. Preheat the oven to 350 degrees F. Lightly, grease a small baking dish.

2. In a large bowl, add eggs, salt and black pepper and beat well.

3. Add carrot and zucchini and stir to combine.

4. Transfer the mixture into prepared baking dish evenly.

5. Bake for about 40 minutes.

Green Garden Quiche (4 servings, serving: 1 portion)

Per Serving, Calories: 116 - Fat: 7.1g - Carbs: 4.3g - Protein: 9.4g

Ingredients:

- 6 organic eggs

- ½ cup of unsweetened almond milk

- Sea salt and freshly ground black pepper, to taste

- 1 cup of chopped fresh baby spinach

- 1 cup of chopped fresh baby kale

- ½ cup of seeded and chopped green bell pepper

- 1 chopped scallion

- ¼ cup of chopped fresh cilantro

- 1 tbsp. of minced fresh chives

Directions:

1. Preheat the oven to 400 degrees F. Lightly grease a pie dish.

2. In a large bowl, add eggs, almond milk, salt and black pepper and beat well. Keep aside.

3. In another bowl, add remaining ingredients. Place the veggie mixture in the bottom of prepared pie dish.

4. Place egg mixture over vegetable mixture evenly.

5. Bake for about 20 minutes or till a toothpick inserted in the center comes out clean.

6. Remove from oven and keep aside to cool for about 5-10 minutes before slicing.

7. Serve warm.

Delish Breakfast Skillet (4 servings, serving: 1 portion)

Per Serving, Calories: 171- Fat: 12.3g - Carbs: 9.2g - Protein: 8.3g

Ingredients:

- 2 tbsp. of olive oil, divided

- 1 pound of quartered and thinly sliced zucchini

- 1 seeded and chopped large red bell pepper

- 1 chopped medium onion

- 1 tsp. of chopped fresh rosemary

- Sea salt, to taste

- 4 large organic eggs

- Freshly ground black pepper, to taste

Directions:

1. In a large skillet, heat 1 tbsp. of oil on medium-high heat.

2. Add zucchini, bell pepper and onion and sauté for about 5-8 minutes.

3. Stir in rosemary and a little salt.

4. With a wooden spoon, make a large well in the center of skillet by moving the veggie mixture towards the sides.

5. Reduce the heat to medium.

6. Pour remaining oil in the well.

7. Carefully, crack the eggs in the well and sprinkle with salt and black pepper.

8. Cook for about 1-2 minutes.

9. Cover the skillet and cook for about 1-2 minutes more.

10. For serving, carefully, scoop the veggie mixture in 4 serving plates. Top with an egg and serve.

Comforting Breakfast (2 servings, serving: 1 portion)

Per Serving, Calories: 177- Fat: 12g - Carbs: 11.7g - Protein: 9.6g

Ingredients:

- 1 tbsp. of olive oil

- 1 minced garlic clove

- 2 spiralized with blade C large zucchinis

- Sea salt and freshly ground black pepper, to taste

- 2 organic eggs

Directions:

1. In a large skillet, heat oil on medium heat.

2. Add garlic and sauté for about 1 minute.

3. Add zucchini, salt and black pepper and cook for about 3-4 minutes.

4. Transfer the zucchini mixture into 2 large serving plates.

5. Meanwhile in a large pan, bring 2-3-inch of water to a boil on medium heat.

6. Carefully, crack the eggs in water, one by one and cook for about 3-4 minutes or till desired doneness.

7. Divide the zucchini mixture in serving plates.

8. Top each plate with 1 egg and sprinkle black pepper and serve.

Nourishing Breakfast Hash (4 servings, serving: 1 portion)

Per Serving, Calories: 92- Fat: 3.7g - Carbs: 14.4g - Protein: 1.6g

Ingredients:

- 1 tbsp. of olive oil

- 1 chopped medium onion

- 1 scrubbed and cubed into ½-inch size large sweet potato

- 1 seeded and chopped large red bell pepper

- 2 tbsp. of water

- Sea salt and freshly ground black pepper, to taste

- 2 tbsp. of chopped scallion (green part)

- 2 tbsp. of minced fresh cilantro

Directions

1. In a large skillet, heat oil on medium heat.

2. Add onion and sauté for about 3-4 minutes.

3. Add sweet potato and cook for about 4-5 minutes, stirring occasionally.

4. Stir in bell pepper and cook for about 1 minute.

5. Add water, sea salt and black pepper and mix well.

6. Cook, covered for about 15-20 minutes, stirring occasionally.

7. Stir in scallion and cilantro and immediately remove from heat.

8. Serve hot.

Amazing Holiday Salad (5 servings, serving: 1 plate)

Per Serving, Calories: 279- Fat: 11.7g - Carbs: 45g - Protein: 2.7g

Ingredients:

For Salad:

- 3 cored and sliced large apples

- ½ cup of fresh cranberries

- 6 cups of fresh baby spinach

- 3 tbsp. of chopped walnuts

For Dressing:

- 3 tbsp. of extra-virgin olive oil

- 2 tbsp. of honey

- 3 tbsp. of fresh apple juice

- 2 tbsp. of apple cider vinegar

Directions:

In a large bowl, mix together all salad ingredients.

In another bowl, add all dressing ingredients and beat till well combined.

Pour dressing over salad and toss to coat well.

Serve immediately.

Tropical Salad (4 servings, serving: 1 plate)

Per Serving, Calories: 131- Fat: 0.8g - Carbs: 32.1g - Protein: 2.1g

Ingredients:

- 1½ cups of peeled and chopped fresh pineapple

- 1½ cups of peeled, pitted and cubed mango

- 8 cups of torn lettuce

- ¼ cup of fresh cranberries

- ¼ cup of chopped fresh mint leaves

- 2 tbsp. of fresh orange juice

- Sea salt and freshly ground black pepper, to taste

Directions:

1. In a large serving bowl, add all ingredients except almonds and toss to coat well.

2. Cover and refrigerate to chill before serving.

3. Serve immediately.

Favorite Autumn Salad (8 servings, serving: 1 plate)

Per Serving, Calories: 155- Fat: 9.5g - Carbs: 15.2g - Protein: 5.6g

Ingredients:

For Dressing:

- 1 minced garlic clove

- 1 tbsp. of minced shallot

- ¼ cup of fresh lemon juice

- ¼ cup of extra-virgin olive oil

- Sea salt and freshly ground black pepper, to taste

For Salad:

- 1½ pound of trimmed and thinly sliced fresh Tuscan kale

- 14-ounce of trimmed and finely grated Brussels sprout

- ½ cup of toasted and chopped almonds

Directions:

1. In a bowl, add all dressing ingredients and beat till well combined.

2. In a large bowl, mix together all salad ingredients.

3. Pour dressing over salad and toss to coat well.

4. Serve immediately.

Warm Tofu Salad (4 servings, serving: 1 plate)

Per Serving, Calories: 180- Fat: 11.5g - Carbs: 12.9g - Protein: 10.6g

Ingredients:

For Dressing:

- 2 tbsp. of balsamic vinegar

- 2 tbsp. of extra-virgin olive oil

- 1 tbsp. of honey

- 1 tsp. of low-sodium tamari

- Sea salt and freshly ground black pepper, to taste

For Salad:

- 1 (14-ounce) package of pressed and cubed extra firm tofu

- 1 peeled and chopped large carrot

- 1 chopped large cucumber

- 8 cups of fresh baby spinach

Directions:

1. In a large bowl, add all dressing ingredients and beat till well combined.

2. In a nonstick skillet, mix together 2 tbsp. of dressing and tofu on medium-high heat.

3. Cook for about 12-15 minutes, flipping after every 2-3 minutes.

4. Remove the skillet from heat and immediately stir in 1 tbsp. of dressing.

5. In a large serving bowl, add cucumber, carrot and spinach.

6. Pour dressing and toss to coat well.

7. Top with warm tofu and serve immediately.

Vibrant Summer Salad (6 servings, serving: 1 plate)

Per Serving, Calories: 97- Fat: 6.5g - Carbs: 9.4g - Protein: 2.7g

Ingredients:

For Salad:

- ¾ pound of trimmed fresh green beans

- 2 cups of halved cherry tomatoes

- 6 cups of torn Bib lettuce

- 2 tbsp. of chopped fresh parsley

- 2 tbsp. of chopped fresh mint leaves

- 2 tbsp. of toasted and chopped walnuts

For Dressing:

- 1 minced shallot

- 1 tbsp. of balsamic vinegar

- Sea salt and freshly ground black pepper, to taste

- 2 tbsp. of extra-virgin olive oil

Directions:

1. In a large pan of boiling water, add green beans and cook for about 4-6 minutes.

2. Drain well and rinse under cold water. With a paper towel pat dry the beans completely.

3. Transfer the beans into a large salad bowl.

4. Meanwhile for dressing in a bowl, add all ingredients except oil and beat well.

5. Slowly, add oil, beating continuously until well combined.

6. Add tomatoes, lettuce and parsley in serving bowl with beans and mix.

7. Pour dressing over salad and toss to coat well.   Top with walnuts and serve.

Nutrient-Filled Soup (8 servings, serving: 1 bowl)

Per Serving, Calories: 92- Fat: 4.5g - Carbs: 12.1g - Protein: 4.2g

Ingredients:

- 2 tbsp. of extra-virgin olive oil

- 1 chopped large onion

- Pinch of sea salt

- 2 sliced large leeks

- 2 tbsp. of minced fresh ginger

- 1 chopped bunch of collard greens

- 8 cups of fat-free, low-sodium vegetable broth

- 1 tbsp. of fresh lemon juice

Directions:

1. In a large soup pan, heat oil on low heat.

2. Add onion and salt and cook for about 20 minutes.

3. Stir in leeks and cook for about 10 minutes.

4. Stir in ginger and greens and cook for about 5 minutes.

5. Add broth and bring to a boil on medium heat.

6. Cook for about 10 minutes.

7. Remove from heat and keep aside to cool slightly.

8. In a blender, add the soup mixture in batches and pulse till smooth.

9. Return the soup in pan on medium heat and cook for about 5 minutes.

10. Stir in lemon juice and serve hot.

Garden Green Soup (4 servings, serving: 1 bowl)

Per Serving, Calories: 205- Fat: 14g - Carbs: 17.4g - Protein: 6.9g

Ingredients:

- 1 tbsp. of extra-virgin olive oil

- 1 chopped small white onion

- 1 chopped celery stalk

- 2 minced garlic cloves

- ¼ tsp. of grated fresh ginger

- 1 tsp. of ground turmeric

- ½ tsp. of ground cumin

- 1/8 tsp. of cayenne pepper

- 1 cut into florets large head of broccoli

- 5 cups of fat-free, low-sodium vegetable broth

- Freshly ground black pepper, to taste

- 1 peeled, pitted and chopped small avocado

- 1 tbsp. of fresh lemon juice

Directions:

1. In a large pan, heat the oil n medium heat.

2. Add onion and celery and sauté for about 4-5 minutes.

3. Add garlic, ginger, turmeric, cumin and cayenne pepper and sauté for about 1 minute.

4. Add broccoli florets, broth and black pepper and bring to a boil.

5. Reduce the heat to medium-low and simmer, covered for about 25-30 minutes.

6. Remove from heat and stir in avocado.

7. With an immersion blender, blend the soup till smooth.

8. Serve immediately with the drizzling f lemon juice.

Velvety Soup (5 servings, serving: 1 bowl)

Per Serving, Calories: 177- Fat: 14.5g - Carbs: 11.1g - Protein: 3.7g

Ingredients:

- 1 tbsp. of extra-virgin olive oil

- 1 chopped yellow onion

- 2 peeled and chopped carrots

- 2 chopped celery stalks

- 2 minced garlic cloves

- 1 finely chopped Serrano pepper

- 1 tsp. of ground turmeric

- 1 tsp. of ground coriander

- 1 tsp. of ground cumin

- ¼ tsp. of crushed red pepper flakes

- 1 chopped head of cauliflower

- 4 cups of fat-free, low-sodium vegetable broth

- 1 cup of unsweetened coconut milk

- Freshly ground black pepper, to taste

- 2 tbsp. of chopped fresh cilantro

Directions:

1. In a large soup pan, heat oil on medium heat.

2. Add onion, carrot and celery and sauté for about 4-5 minutes.

3. Add garlic, Serrano pepper and spices and sauté for about 1 minute.

4. Add cauliflower and cook, stirring often for about 5 minutes.

5. Add broth and coconut milk and bring to a boil on medium-high heat.

6. Reduce the heat to low and simmer for about 15 minutes or till desired doneness of vegetables.

7. Season the soup with black pepper and remove from heat.

8. Serve hot with the topping of cilantro.

Distinctive Veggie Soup (4 servings, serving: 1 bowl)

Per Serving, Calories: 157- Fat: 3.8g - Carbs: 27.9g - Protein: 3.9g

Ingredients:

- 1 tbsp. of extra-virgin olive oil

- 1 sliced shallot

- 1 chopped onion

- 2 minced garlic cloves

- 1 tsp. of paprika

- 3 peeled and cubed sweet potatoes

- Freshly ground black pepper, to taste

- 4 cups of fat-free, low-sodium vegetable broth

Directions:

1. In a large soup pan, heat oil on medium heat.

2. Add shallot and onion and sauté for about 4-5 minutes.

3. Add garlic and paprika sauté for about 1 minute.

4. Add sweet potatoes, black pepper and broth and bring to a boil.

5. Reduce the heat to low and simmer for about 25-30 minutes.

6. Remove from heat and let it cool slightly.

7. In a blender, add soup in batches and pulse till smooth.

8. Return the soup in the pan and cook for 3-4 minutes or till heated completely.

9. Serve hot.

Aromatic Soup (6 servings, serving: 1 bowl)

Per Serving, Calories: 71- Fat: 4.9g - Carbs: 5.5g - Protein: 2g

Ingredients:

- 2 tbsp. of canola oil

- 1½ cups of chopped onion

- 2 minced garlic cloves

- ½ tsp. of crushed dried thyme

- 2 cups of finely chopped tomatoes

- 2 tsp. balsamic vinegar

- 6 cups of fat-free, low-sodium vegetable broth

- ¼ cup of chopped fresh basil leaves

- Sea salt and freshly ground black pepper, to taste

Directions:

1. In a large soup pan, heat oil on medium heat.

2. Add onion and sauté for about 4-5 minutes.

3. Add garlic and thyme and sauté for about 1 minute.

4. Add tomatoes, vinegar and broth and bring to a boil.

5. Reduce the heat to low and simmer, covered for about 15 minutes.

6. Remove from heat and keep aside to cool slightly.

7. In a blender, add soup in batches and pulse till smooth.

8. Return the soup in the pan. Stir in basil and cook for about 3-4 minutes.

9. Season with salt and black pepper and serve hot.

Hearty Lettuce Wraps (4 servings, serving: 2 wraps)

Per Serving, Calories: 183- Fat: 3.9g - Carbs: 30.4g - Protein: 7.9g

Ingredients:

For Filling:

- 1 tsp. of olive oil

- 2 cups of chopped fresh shiitake mushrooms

- 2 tsp. of low-sodium tamari, divided

- 1 cup of cooked quinoa

- 2 tsp. of fresh lime juice

- ¼ cup of chopped scallion

- Freshly ground black pepper, to taste

For Wraps:

- 8 medium butter lettuce leaves

- ¼ cup of peeled and julienned cucumber

- ¼ cup of peeled and julienned carrot

Directions:

1. For filling in a skillet, heat oil on medium heat.

2. Add mushrooms and 1 tsp. of low-sodium tamari and cook for about 5-8 minutes.

3. Stir on quinoa, lime juice and remaining low-sodium tamari and cook for about 1` minute.

4. Stir in scallion, black pepper and immediately, remove from heat. Keep aside to cool.

5. Place lettuce leaves into serving plates.

6. Place quinoa filling over each leaf evenly.

7. Top with cucumber and carrot and serve.

Asian Style Lettuce Wraps (4 servings, serving: 2 wraps)

Per Serving, Calories: 166- Fat: 7.3g - Carbs: 6.91g - Protein: 18.8g

Ingredients:

- 2 tsp. of olive oil

- 1 cup of chopped onion

- ¾ pound of grass-fed lean ground chicken

- 1 cup of chopped fresh mushrooms

- ½ tbsp. of minced fresh ginger

- 1 tbsp. of low-sodium tamari

- ½ tbsp. of cayenne pepper

- ½ tbsp. of ground cumin

- 8 romaine lettuce leaves

- 1 peeled and julienned large carrot

- 2 tbsp. of chopped fresh cilantro leaves

Directions:

1. In a skillet, heat oil on medium heat.

2. Add onion and sauté for about 4-5 minutes.

3. Add chicken and cook for about 6-8 minutes, stirring occasionally.

4. Add mushroom, ginger, low-sodium tamari, cayenne pepper and cumin and cook for about 4 minutes.

5. Remove from heat and keep aside.

6. Meanwhile in a bowl, mix together all sauce ingredients.

7. Arrange the lettuce leaves in serving plates.

8. Place turkey mixture over each lettuce leaf evenly.

9. Top with carrot and cilantro evenly and serve.

Flavor-Packed Burgers (4 servings, serving: 1 burger with 1 portion kale)

Per Serving, Calories: 386- Fat: 8.8g - Carbs: 63.1g - Protein: 18.6g

Ingredients:

- 1 tbsp. of olive oil, divided

- 1 finely chopped small onion

- 1½ cups of cooked chickpeas

- 1 peeled and chopped carrot

- ½ cup of chopped fresh parsley

- 2 minced garlic cloves

- 1 chopped jalapeño pepper

- ½ cup of whole wheat bread crumbs

- ¼ tsp. of ground cumin

- ¼ tsp. of ground coriander

- Sea salt, to taste

- 6 cups of fresh baby kale

Directions

1. Preheat oven to 400 degrees. Lightly grease a baking sheet.

2. In a small nonstick pan, heat ½ tbsp. of olive oil on medium heat.

3. Add onion and sauté for about 5 minutes.

4. Remove from heat and transfer into a large bowl.

5. In a food processor, add chickpeas, carrot, parsley, garlic and jalapeño pepper and pulse till smooth.

6. Transfer the chickpea mixture into bowl with onion and mix well.

7. Add bread crumbs, cumin, coriander and cumin and salt and mix till well combined.

8. Make 4 (½-inch thick) patties from the mixture.

9. Coat the patties with remaining olive oil evenly and arrange onto the prepared baking sheet in a single layer.

10. Bake for about 15-20 minutes or till top becomes golden brown.

11. Divide kale into 4 serving plates.

12. Place 1 patty in each plate and serve.

Awesome Burgers (8 servings, serving: 1 burger with 1 portion salad)

Per Serving, Calories: 223- Fat: 14.2g - Carbs: 17.5g - Protein: 7.2g

Ingredients:

- 1 cup of water

- ½ cup of red quinoa

- 1 tbsp. of canola oil

- 1 cup of chopped onion

- 2 cups of finely chopped white button mushrooms

- 1 tsp. of minced garlic

- ¾ tsp. of crushed dried marjoram

- ¼ tsp. of crushed dried oregano

- 2/3 cup of shredded low-fat Cheddar cheese

- 1 beaten large organic egg

- ½ cup of toasted and finely chopped pecans

- 1/3 cup of quick-cooking rolled oats

- 1 tbsp. of low-sodium tamari

- 12 cups of torn lettuce

Directions:

1. In a medium pan, add water and quinoa and bring to a boil.

2. Reduce the heat to low and simmer, covered and for about 15 minutes.

3. Remove from heat and keep aside, covered for about 10 minutes.

4. With a fork, fluff the quinoa and keep aside to cool.

5. Preheat oven to 350 degrees F. Lightly grease a baking sheet.

6. In a large pan, heat oil on medium heat.

7. Add onion and sauté for about 5 minutes.

8. Add mushrooms, garlic and herbs and cook for about 5 minutes, stirring continuously.

9. Remove from the heat and keep aside to cool for about 5 minutes.

10. In a bowl, add quinoa, mushroom mixture, cheese, egg, pecans, oats and tamari and stir to combine well.

11. Make 8 equal sized patties from the mixture.

12. Arrange the patties onto the prepared baking sheet in a single layer.

13. Bake for about 28-30 minutes or till top becomes golden brown.

14. Divide lettuce into 8 serving plates.

15. Place 1 patty in each plate and serve.

Foolproof Burgers (6 servings, serving: 1 burger with 1 portion arugula)

Per Serving, Calories: 287- Fat: 9.8g - Carbs: 36.9g - Protein: 15.8g

Ingredients:

- 1¾ cups plus 1 tbsp. of water

- ¾ cup of rinsed and strained brown lentils

- 2 tsp. of extra-virgin olive oil

- ½ of finely chopped large red onion

- 1 tbsp. of fresh lemon juice

- Sea salt, to taste

- 8-ounce of fresh baby spinach

- 2 minced large garlic cloves

- Freshly ground black pepper, to taste

- ½ tsp. of ground cumin

- 1 cup of whole-wheat breadcrumbs

- ½ cup of toasted and finely chopped walnuts

- Cooking spray

- 10 cups of fresh baby arugula

Directions:

1. In a pan, add 1¾ cups of water and lentils on high heat and bring to a boil.

2. Reduce the heat to medium-low and simmer, covered partially for about 30 minutes.

3. Transfer the lentils into a bowl.

4. Add remaining 1 tbsp. of water and with a potato masher, mash well.

5. In a large nonstick skillet, heat oil on medium heat.

6. Add onion, lemon juice and a pinch of salt and sauté for about 6 minutes.

7. Add spinach, garlic, cumin and black pepper and cook for about 3 minutes.

8. Transfer the spinach mixture into the bowl with mashed lentils.

9. Add breadcrumbs, walnuts and salt and mix till well combined.

10. Refrigerate, covered for at least 1 hour or overnight.

11. Preheat the grill to medium-high heat and lightly, grease the grill grate.

12. Make 6 (4-inch) patties from the mixture.

13. Coat the patties with the cooking spray from both sides.

14. Grill the patties for about 3 minutes per side.

15. Divide the arugula into 6 serving plates.

16. Place 1 patty in each plate and serve.

Classic Burgers (2 servings, serving: 1 burger with 1 portion salad)

Per Serving, Calories: 189- Fat: 9.1g - Carbs: 14.1g - Protein: 14.7g

Ingredients:

- ¼ pound of lean grass-fed ground chicken

- 1 tbsp. of crumbled low-fat feta cheese

- 1 minced garlic clove

- 1½ tsp. of chopped fresh parsley

- Sea salt and freshly ground black pepper

- 2 tsp. of olive oil, divided

- 8 tomato slices

- 1 sliced red onion

- 3 cups of fresh baby greens

Directions:

1. In a bowl, add chicken, cheese, garlic, parsley, salt and pepper and mix till well combined.

2. Make 2 patties from the mixture.

3. In a frying pan, heat 1 tsp. of oil on medium heat.

4. Add patties and cook for about 6-8 minutes per side.

5. Meanwhile in another frying pan, heat remaining oil on medium heat.

6. Cook tomato and onion slices for about 1-2 minutes per side.

7. Divide the greens, tomato slices and onion slices into 2 serving plates.

8. Place 1 patty in each plate and serve.

Super-Tasty Meatballs (8 servings, serving: 1 portion meatballs & salad)

Per Serving, Calories: 230- Fat: 8.3g - Carbs: 23.2g - Protein: 17.9g

Ingredients:

For Meatballs:

- 1 pound of lean ground turkey

- 1 cup of cooked and roughly mashed black beans

- 1 seeded and finely chopped small red bell pepper

- 1 seeded and finely chopped small yellow bell pepper

- ½ cup of chopped fresh parsley

- Sea salt and freshly ground black pepper, to taste

- 2 tbsp. of olive oil

For Serving:

- 10 cups of shredded lettuce leaves

- 4 cups of halved cherry tomatoes

Directions:

1. For meatballs in a large bowl, add all ingredients and mix till well combined.

2. Make equal sized 24 balls from mixture.

3. In a skillet, heat oil on medium heat.

4. Add meatballs and cook for about 5-7 minutes or till golden brown from all sides.

5. Cover the skillet and cook for about 5 minutes more.

6. Divide lettuce and cherry tomatoes in 12 serving plates.

7. Place 3 meatballs in each plate and serve.

Popular Winter Lunch (3 servings, serving: 1 portion)

Per Serving, Calories: 164- Fat: 3.4g - Carbs: 32.1g - Protein: 2g

Ingredients:

- 2 tsp. of olive oil

- 1 chopped onion

- 2 peeled and cubed medium sweet potatoes

- ½ tbsp. of ground turmeric

- 1 tsp. of chopped fresh parsley

- Sea salt and freshly ground black pepper, to taste

- Water, as required

Directions:

1. In a skillet, heat oil on low heat.

2. Add onion and sauté for about 8-10 minutes.

3. Stir in sweet potato turmeric, parsley, salt and black pepper.

4. Add enough water to covers the sweet potato half way.

5. Cook for about 6-8 minutes or till desired doneness.

Ideal Luncheon Meal (4 servings, serving: 1 portion)

Per Serving, Calories: 124- Fat: 7.9g - Carbs: 12.9g - Protein: 4.5g

Ingredients:

- 2 tbsp. of olive oil

- 1 tbsp. of minced fresh ginger

- 1 tbsp. of minced garlic

- 1 tbsp. of cumin seeds

- 1 tsp. of smoked paprika

- Sea salt and freshly ground black pepper, to taste

- 1 pound of trimmed and halved Brussels sprouts

- ½ cup of water

Directions:

1. In a skillet, heat oil on medium heat.

2. Add ginger and garlic and sauté for about 2 minutes.

3. Add cumin seeds, paprika, salt and black pepper and sauté for about 2 minutes.

4. Add Brussels sprouts and water and stir to combine.

5. Cook, covered for about 6-8 minutes.

6. Serve hot.

Fuss-Free Lunch (2 servings, serving: 1 portion)

Per Serving, Calories: 138- Fat: 13g - Carbs: 4.6g - Protein: 3g

Ingredients:

- 1 tbsp. of olive oil

- 2 minced garlic cloves

- ½ pound of trimmed fresh green beans

- Sea salt and freshly ground black pepper, to taste

- ½ cup of water

- ¼ cup of toasted and slivered almonds

Directions:

1. In a skillet, heat oil on medium heat.

2. Add garlic and sauté for about 1 minute.

3. Add green beans and cook for about 4-5 minutes.

4. Add water and bring to a boil.

5. Cook, covered for about 10 minutes.

6. Add salt, black pepper and almond and toss to coat.

7. Serve hot.

Healthy Veggie Combo (4 servings, serving: 1 portion)

Per Serving, Calories: 94- Fat: 7.4g - Carbs: 6.4g - Protein: 3.1g

Ingredients:

- ½ tbsp. of fresh ginger paste

- ½ tbsp. of garlic paste

- 1 tsp. of ground cumin

- Sea salt and freshly ground black pepper, to taste

- 2 tbsp. of olive oil, divided

- 1 pound of trimmed and cut into 1-inch pieces asparagus

- ½ cup of broccoli florets

- 2 tbsp. of fresh lemon juice

Directions:

1. In a bowl, mix together, ginger, garlic paste, cumin, salt, black pepper and 1 tsp. oil.

2. Add asparagus and broccoli and toss to coat well.

3. In a large skillet, heat remaining oil on medium heat.

4. Add onion and sauté for about 2 minutes.

5. Add asparagus mixture and stir fry for about 5 minutes.

6. Stir in lemon juice and remove from heat.

Flavor-Packed Broccoli (2 servings, serving: 1 portion)

Per Serving, Calories: 192- Fat: 12.3g - Carbs: 19.1g - Protein: 5.4g

Ingredients:

- 8-ounce of chopped broccoli

- 1 tbsp. of canola oil

- 1 chopped onion

- 2 chopped tomatoes

- ¼ tsp. of ground turmeric

- ¼ tsp, of ground cumin

- ½ tsp. ground coriander

- 1 tbsp. of shredded coconut

- ¼ cup of water

- 2 tbsp. of unsweetened coconut milk

- 1 tbsp. of fresh lemon juice

Directions:

1. In a pan of boiling water, arrange a steamer basket.

2. Place the broccoli in steamer basket and steam, covered for about 5 minutes. Drain well.

3. In a skillet, heat oil on medium heat.

4. Add onion and sauté for about 5 minutes.

5. Add remaining ingredients and bring to a gentle simmer.

6. Stir in broccoli and simmer for about 5 minutes.

7. Serve hot.

Glazed Carrots (4 servings, serving: 1 portion)

Per Serving, Calories: 113- Fat: 3.5g - Carbs: 20.9g - Protein: 1g

Ingredients:

- 1 cup of water

- 1 pound of peeled and cut into ½-inch slices carrot

- Sea salt, to taste

- 1 tbsp. olive oil

- 2 tsp. of finely grated fresh orange zest

- 2 tbsp. of honey

- 2 tbsp. of fresh orange juice

- Freshly ground black pepper, to taste

Directions:

1. In a pan, add water, carrots and a pinch of salt and bring to a boil on high heat.

2. Reduce the heat to medium and simmer for about 5 minutes.

3. Drain the water well.

4. In the same pan, add remaining ingredients and carrot on medium heat and sauté for about 2-3 minutes or till glaze becomes slightly thick.

5. Serve hot.

South-Asian Favorite Luncheon (4 servings, serving: 1 portion)

Per Serving, Calories: 131- Fat: 7.6g - Carbs: 14g - Protein: 4.1g

Ingredients:

- ¼ cup of water

- 2 chopped medium fresh tomatoes

- 2 tbsp. of olive oil

- 1 chopped small onion

- ½ tbsp. of minced fresh ginger

- 3 minced garlic cloves

- 1 seeded and chopped jalapeño pepper

- 1 tsp. of ground cumin

- 1 tsp. of ground coriander

- 1 tsp. of cayenne pepper

- ¼ tsp. of ground turmeric

- 2 cups of chopped cauliflower

- 1 cup of shelled fresh green peas

- Sea salt and freshly ground black pepper, to taste

- ½ cup of warm water

- ¼ cup of chopped fresh cilantro leaves

Directions:

1. In a blender, add ¼ cup of water and tomatoes and pulse till pureed. Keep aside.

2. In a large skillet, heat oil on medium heat.

3. Add onion and sauté for about 4-5 minutes.

4. Add ginger, garlic, ginger, jalapeño pepper and spices and sauté for about 1 minute.

5. Add tomato puree, cauliflower and peas and cook for about 3-4 minutes, stirring continuously.

6. Add warm water and bring to a boil.

7. Reduce the heat to medium-low and simmer, covered for about 8-10 minutes or till desired doneness of vegetables.

8. Serve hot with the garnishing of cilantro.

Garlicky Spinach (3 servings, serving: 1 portion)

Per Serving, Calories: 81- Fat: 5.1g - Carbs: 8.1g - Protein: 2.6g

Ingredients:

- 1 tbsp. of olive oil

- 1 finely chopped red onion

- 6 minced garlic cloves

- ½ tsp. of minced fresh ginger

- 1 tsp. of ground coriander

- ½ tsp. of ground cumin

- ¼ tsp. of ground turmeric

- 6 cups of chopped fresh spinach

- Sea salt and freshly ground black pepper, to taste

- 1-2 tbsp. of water

Directions:

1. In a large skillet, melt coconut oil on medium heat.

2. Add onion and sauté for about 8 minutes.

3. Add garlic, ginger and spices and sauté for about 1 minute.

4. Add spinach, salt and black pepper and cook for about 2 minutes, stirring occasionally.

5. Add water and cook for about 3 minutes.

6. Cook, covered for about 15 minutes.

7. Uncover and stir fry for about 2 minutes.

8. Serve warm.

Strengthening Meal (4 servings, serving: 1 portion)

Per Serving, Calories: 134- Fat: 7.3g - Carbs: 15.7g - Protein: 4g

Ingredients:

- 2 tbsp. of extra-virgin olive oil

- 1 chopped yellow onion

- 2 chopped garlic cloves

- ½ teaspoon of crushed red pepper flakes

- ¼ tsp. of ground turmeric

- 2 trimmed and chopped bunches fresh kale

- Freshly ground black pepper, to taste

- 2 cups of chopped tomatoes

- ¾ cup of fat-free, low-sodium vegetable broth

Directions:

1. In a large pan, heat oil on medium-high heat.

2. Add onion and sauté for about 4 minutes.

3. Add garlic, red pepper flakes and turmeric and sauté for about 1 minute.

4. Add kale and black pepper and cook for about 2 minutes.

5. Stir in tomatoes and cook for about 1 minute.

6. Add broth and bring to a gentle boil.

7. Reduce the heat to medium and cook, covered for about 15 minutes.

Super-Food Luncheon (2 servings, serving: 1 portion)

Per Serving, Calories: 211- Fat: 14.6g - Carbs: 18g - Protein: 6.8g

Ingredients:

- 2 tbsp. of extra-virgin olive oil, divided

- 4 minced garlic cloves

- ½ of finely chopped red onion

- 1 bunch of trimmed and chopped fresh kale

- Water, as required

- 1 bunch of chopped fresh spinach

- Sea salt and freshly ground black pepper, to taste

Directions:

1. In a large nonstick skillet, heat 2 tbsp. of oil on medium-low heat.

2. Add garlic and sauté for about 1 minute.

3. Add onion and a pinch of salt sauté for about 4-5 minutes.

4. Add kale and a few tsp. of water and increase the heat to medium.

5. Cook, covered for about 2-3 minutes.

6. Stir in spinach and 1-2 tsp. of water and cook, covered for about 5-8 minutes.

7. Stir in remaining oil and increase the heat to medium-high.

8. Stir fry for about 3-4 minutes.

9. Stir in sat and black pepper and remove from heat.

10. Serve hot.

Divine Veggie Pasta (4 servings, serving: 1 portion)

Per Serving, Calories: 210- Fat: 19.6g - Carbs: 8.6g - Protein: 2.2g

Ingredients:

- 1½ tbsp. of canola oil

- ¼ cup of chopped onion

- 2 minced garlic cloves

- 1 finely chopped jalapeño pepper

- 1 peeled and spiralized large carrot

- 1 spiralized large yellow squash

- 1 spiralized large zucchini

- 2 tbsp. of fresh lemon juice

- Sea salt and freshly ground black pepper, to taste

- ½ cup of chopped scallion

Directions:

1. In a large skillet, heat oil on medium heat.

2. Add onion and sauté for about 4-5 minutes.

3. Add garlic and jalapeño pepper and sauté for about 1 minute.

4. Add carrot and cook for about 2-3 minutes.

5. Add squash and zucchini and cook for about 3-4 minutes.

6. Stir in lemon juice, salt and black pepper and remove from heat.

7. Serve immediately with the garnishing of scallion.

Super Healthy Lunch (4 servings, serving: 1 portion)

Per Serving, Calories: 110- Fat: 3.9g - Carbs: 19.7g - Protein: 1.8g

Ingredients:

- 1 tbsp. of extra-virgin olive oil, divided

- 2 minced garlic cloves

- 1 seeded and minced Serrano pepper

- 2 cups of small broccoli florets

- ½ cup of chopped celery stalk

- ¼ cup of fat-free low-sodium vegetable broth

- 2 cored and sliced apples

Directions:

1. In a large skillet, heat oil on medium-high heat.

2. Add garlic and Serrano pepper and sauté for about 1 minute.

3. Add broccoli and stir fry for about 4-5 minutes.

4. Add celery and onion and stir fry for about 4-5 minutes.

5. Stir in broth and cook for about 2-3 minutes.

6. Stir in apple slices and cook for about 2-3 minutes.

7. Serve hot.

Refreshingly Tasty Meal (4 servings, serving: 1 portion)

Per Serving, Calories: 168- Fat: 4g - Carbs: 32.6g - Protein: 3.4g

Ingredients:

For Sauce:

- 1 tbsp. of finely grated fresh orange zest

- 1 tsp. of minced fresh ginger

- 2 minced garlic cloves

- ½ cup of fresh orange juice

- 2 tbsp. of low-sodium tamari

- 2 tbsp. of balsamic vinegar

For Apples & Vegetables:

- 1 tbsp. of olive oil

- 1 chopped Serrano pepper

- 2 cups of cut into small florets broccoli

- 2 cups of peeled and julienned carrot

- 1 cup of chopped onion

- 1 cup of chopped celery

- 2 cored and sliced apples

Directions:

1. In a large bowl, mix together all sauce ingredients. Keep aside.

2. In a large skillet, heat oil on medium-high heat.

3. Add Serrano pepper and sauté for about 30 seconds.

4. Add broccoli and carrot and stir fry for about 4-5 minutes.

5. Add onion and celery and stir fry for about 4-5 minutes.

6. Stir in sauce and cook for about 2-3 minutes, stirring occasionally.

7. Stir in apple slices and cook for about 2-3 minutes more.

8. Serve hot.

Fabulous Tofu (2 servings, serving: 1 portion)

Per Serving, Calories: 181- Fat: 3.7g - Carbs: 6.2g - Protein: 12.2g

Ingredients:

- 1 tbsp. of extra-virgin olive oil, divided

- 8-ounce of drained and cubed extra-firm tofu

- 4 sliced scallions

- 1 tsp. of low-sodium tamari

- 3 roughly chopped garlic cloves

Directions:

1. In a nonstick skillet, heat oil on medium-high heat.

2. Add tofu and cook for about 3 minutes per side.

3. Transfer the tofu into a plate.

4. In the same skillet, add garlic and sauté for about 30 seconds.

5. Add tamari and stir fry for about 30 seconds.

6. Stir in cooked tofu and scallions and stir fry for about 1-2 minutes.

7. Serve hot.

Irresistible Luncheon (3 servings, serving: 1 portion)

Per Serving, Calories: 209- Fat: 13.7g - Carbs: 15.7g - Protein: 11.1g

Ingredients:

- 1½ tbsp. of extra-virgin olive oil, divided
- 8-ounce of pressed and cut into 1-inch slices extra-firm tofu
- 2 thinly sliced garlic cloves
- ¼ cup of toasted and chopped pecans
- 1 tbsp. of honey
- ¼ cup of chopped fresh cilantro
- Pinch of sea salt
- ½ pound of cut into wide ribbons Brussels sprouts

Directions:

1. In a skillet, heat ½ tbsp. of oil on medium heat.
2. Add tofu and sauté for about 4 minutes or till golden brown from all sides.
3. Add garlic and pecans, and sauté for about 1 minute.
4. Add honey and cook for about 2 minutes.
5. Remove from heat and stir in cilantro.
6. Transfer tofu into a plate and keep aside.
7. In the same skillet, heat remaining oil on medium-high heat.
8. Add Brussels sprouts and salt and cook for about 5 minutes.
9. Divide the Brussels sprouts in serving plates.

10. Top with tofu and serve.

Naturally Nutritious Pilaf (3 servings, serving: 1 portion)

Per Serving, Calories: 196- Fat: 8.8g - Carbs: 25.4g - Protein: 4.8g

Ingredients:

- 1½ tbsp. of extra-virgin olive oil, divided

- 1 chopped small onion

- 2 peeled and sliced carrots

- 1 chopped celery stalk

- 1 minced garlic clove

- ½ cup of rinsed and drained quinoa

- 1 cup of water

- 1 tsp. of ground turmeric

- ¼ tsp. of crushed dried basil

- Sea salt, to taste

- 1 tsp. of fresh lemon juice

Directions:

In a large pan, heat oil on medium heat.

Add onion, carrot, celery and garlic and sauté for about 4-5 minutes.

Stir in quinoa, water, turmeric and basil and bring to a gentle boil.

Reduce the heat to low and simmer, covered for about 25-30 minutes or till all the liquid is absorbed.

Stir in salt and lemon juice and remove from heat.

Serve hot.

Amazingly Healthy Pilaf (4 servings, serving: 1 portion)

Per Serving, Calories: 209- Fat: 6.4g - Carbs: 31.1g - Protein: 7.5g

Ingredients:

- 1 tbsp. of extra-virgin olive oil, divided

- 1 tsp. of grated fresh ginger

- 1 tsp. of ground turmeric

- ¼ tsp. of ground coriander

- ¼ tsp. of ground cumin

- 1 cup of rinsed and drained golden quinoa

- 1½ cups of water

- 1½ cups of chopped fresh spinach leaves

- ½ cup of thinly sliced scallions

- ¼ cup of fresh lime juice

- Sea salt and freshly ground black pepper, to taste

Directions:

1. In a medium pan, heat oil on medium-high heat.

2. Add ginger and spices and sauté for about 30 seconds.

3. Add quinoa and stir to combine.

4. Add water and bring to a boil.

5. Reduce the heat and simmer, covered for about15 minutes or till all the liquid is absorbed.

6. Stir in spinach and remove from heat.

7. Keep aside, covered for about 5 minutes. Stir in scallion, lime juice, salt and pepper and serve.

Chapter 3: Dinner Recipes

Colorful Salad (4 servings, serving: 1 plate)

Per Serving, Calories: 226- Fat: 2.7g - Carbs: 46.8g - Protein: 6.6g

Ingredients:

- ¾ cup of rinsed and drained red quinoa

- 1½ tsp. of curry powder

- Freshly ground black pepper, to taste

- 1½ cups of fat-free, low-sodium vegetable broth

- 2 peeled, pitted and cubed medium mangoes

- 3 chopped scallions

Directions:

1. In a pan, add quinoa, garlic powder, curry powder, Sea salt, black pepper and broth on high heat and bring to a boil.

2. Reduce the heat to medium-low and simmer, covered for about 15-20 minutes or till all the liquid is absorbed.

3. Remove from heat and keep covered for about 5 minutes.

4. Uncover and keep aside to cool completely.

5. With a fork, fluff the quinoa.

6. Transfer the quinoa into a large bowl,

7. Add remaining ingredients and stir to combine.

8. Serve immediately.

Greek Style Salad (5 servings, serving: 1 plate)

Per Serving, Calories: 382- Fat: 10.8g - Carbs: 57.6g - Protein: 16.9g

Ingredients:

For Salad:

- 2 cups of cooked chickpeas

- 1 head of shredded butter lettuce

- 1 seeded and chopped orange bell pepper

- 2 cups of halved cherry tomatoes

- 1 chopped red onion

- 3 tbsp. of chopped fresh cilantro leaves

For Dressing:

- 1 seeded and minced Serrano pepper

- 1 minced garlic clove

- 2 tbsp. of extra-virgin olive oil

- 3 tbsp. of balsamic vinegar

- 1 tbsp. of fresh lemon juice

- ¼ tsp. of crushed red pepper flakes

- Sea salt and freshly ground black pepper, to taste

Directions:

1. In a large serving bowl, add all salad ingredients and mix.

2. In another bowl, add all dressing ingredients and beat till well combined.

3. Pour dressing over salad and gently toss to coat well.

4. Serve immediately.

All-in-One Salad (2 servings, serving: 1 plate)

Per Serving, Calories: 306- Fat: 13.7g - Carbs: 21.2g - Protein: 25.4g

Ingredients:

For Salad:

- 1 (6-ounce) cooked and cubed grass-fed chicken breast

- 1 cored and chopped large apple

- 1 chopped medium celery stalk

- ½ shredded head of lettuce

For Dressing:

- 2 tbsp. of olive oil

- 2 tbsp. of fresh lemon juice

- 2 tbsp. of apple cider vinegar

- 1 tsp. of honey

- Sea salt and freshly ground black pepper, to taste

Directions:

1. In a large serving bowl, add all salad ingredients and mix.

2. In another bowl, add all dressing ingredients and beat till well combined.

3. Pour dressing over salad and gently toss to coat well.

4. Serve immediately.

Best-Ever Beef Salad (6 servings, serving: 1 plate)

Per Serving, Calories: 218- Fat: 11.3g - Carbs: 7.4g - Protein: 22.1g

Ingredients:

- 2 tbsp. of fresh lemon juice, divided

- 2 tbsp. of extra-virgin olive oil, divided

- Sea salt and freshly ground black pepper, to taste

- 1 pound of trimmed grass-fed flank steak

- 1 tsp. of honey

- 10 cups of fresh baby arugula

- 4 pitted and thinly sliced plums

Directions:

1. In a large bowl, mix together 1 teaspoon of lemon juice, 1½ teaspoons of extra-virgin olive oil, pinch of salt and black pepper.

2. Add steak and coat with mixture generously.

3. Heat a lightly greased nonstick skillet on medium high-heat.

4. Add beef steak and cook for 5 minutes per side.

5. Transfer the steak onto a cutting board and keep aside for about 10 minutes before slicing.

6. With a sharp knife, cut the beef steak diagonally across grain in desired size slices.

7. In a large bowl, add remaining lemon juice, oil, honey, salt and black pepper and beat well.

8. Add arugula and toss well.

9. Divide arugula in 4 serving plates.

10. Top with beef slices and plum slices evenly and serve.

Warming Soup (8 servings, serving: 1 bowl)

Per Serving, Calories: 175- Fat: 12.1g - Carbs: 15.9g - Protein: 2.6g

Ingredients:

For Soup:

- 4 cups of unsweetened almond milk, divided

- 4 cups of peeled and chopped carrots

- 1 tsp. of ground cumin

- ½ tsp. of ground cinnamon

- 1 tsp. of ground ginger

- 1 tsp. of sweet paprika

- 3 cups of water

- Sea salt and freshly ground black pepper, to taste

For Quinoa:

- ½ cup of quinoa

- 1½ tbsp. of olive oil

- Sea salt, to taste

- 1 tbsp. of honey

Directions:

1. For soup in a large soup pan, add 3 cups of almond milk and remaining ingredients and bring to a boil on high heat.

2. Reduce the heat to medium-low and simmer for about 15-20 minutes.

3. Remove from heat and keep aside to cool slightly.

4. In a blender, add soup in batches and pulse till smooth.

5. Transfer the soup and remaining almond milk in pan and cook for about 2-3 minutes.

6. Remove from heat and transfer into a large bowl.

7. Meanwhile in anther pan of salted boiling water, add quinoa and cook for about 8-10 minutes.

8. Drain well and transfer into a bowl.

9. In a nonstick skillet, heat oil medium heat.

10. Add quinoa, salt and brown sugar and cook, stirring continuously for about 5-7 minutes.

11. Serve the soup with the topping of quinoa.

Beans Soup (8 servings, serving: 1 bowl)

Per Serving, Calories: 320- Fat: 4.6g - Carbs: 53.2g - Protein: 19g

Ingredients:

- 2 tbsp. of canola oil

- 1 chopped large onion

- 8 minced garlic cloves

- 1 tsp. of ground cumin

- 1 tsp. of ground coriander

- 1 tsp. of smoked paprika

- 1/8 tsp. of cayenne pepper

- 22-ounce of cooked kidney beans

- 2 cups of chopped tomatoes

- Freshly ground black pepper, to taste

- 5½ cups of water

- 1 (5-ounce) package of fresh baby spinach

Directions:

1. In a large soup pan, heat oil on medium heat.

2. Add onion and sauté for about 4-5 minutes.

3. Add garlic and spices and sauté for about 1 minute.

4. Add beans, tomatoes, black pepper and water and bring to a boil.

5. Reduce the heat to low and simmer for about 45 minutes.

6. Remove from heat and cool slightly.

7. With a potato masher, blend half of beans

8. Return the soup to pan on medium heat.

9. Stir in spinach and simmer for about 3-4 minutes.

10. Serve hot.

Nutritive Soup (4 servings, serving: 1 bowl)

Per Serving, Calories: 277- Fat: 15.1g - Carbs: 37.7g - Protein: 3.7g

Ingredients:

- 2 tbsp. of canola oil

- 1 chopped small onion

- 1 cup of peeled and chopped carrot

- 4 minced garlic cloves

- ½ tsp. of crushed dried thyme

- ½ tsp. of crushed dried basil

- ½ tsp. of ground cumin

- ¼ tsp. of ground turmeric

- 1 tsp. of crushed red pepper flakes

- ¼ tsp. of cayenne pepper

- 3 cups of peeled, seeded and chopped pumpkin

- 2 cups of peeled, cored and chopped apple

- 4 cups of water

- ½ cup unsweetened coconut milk

- Freshly ground black pepper, to taste

Directions:

1. In a large soup pan, heat oil on medium heat.

2. Add onion and carrot and sauté for about 4-5 minutes.

3. Add garlic, herbs and spices and sauté for about 1 minute.

4. Add pumpkin, apple and broth and bring to a boil on high heat.

5. Reduce the heat to medium-low and simmer, covered for about 30-40 minutes.

6. Remove from heat and keep aside to cool slightly.

7. Transfer the mixture in a high speed blender in batches and pulse till smooth.

8. Return the soup in pan and stir in coconut milk and black pepper.

9. Cook for about 3-4 minutes or till heated completely.

10. Serve hot.

Popular Asian Soup (4 servings, serving: 1 bowl)

Per Serving, Calories: 233- Fat: 11.9g - Carbs: 4.2g - Protein: 27.4g

Ingredients:

- 1 tbsp. of olive oil

- 1 chopped yellow onion

- 1 minced garlic clove

- 4 cups of fat-free, low-sodium chicken broth

- 1 pound of cubed boneless salmon

- 1 tbsp. of low-sodium tamari

- 2 tbsp. of chopped fresh cilantro leaves

- Freshly ground black pepper, to taste

- 1 tbsp. of fresh lime juice

Directions:

1. In a large soup pan, heat oil on medium heat.

2. Add onion and sauté for about 5 minutes.

3. Add garlic and lime leaves and sauté for about 1 minute.

4. Add broth and bring to a boil on high heat.

5. Reduce the heat to low and simmer for about 15 minutes.

6. Add salmon and tamari and cook for about 3-4 minutes.

7. Stir in black pepper, lime juice and cilantro and serve hot.

Thanksgiving Dinner Soup (8 servings, serving: 1 bowl)

Per Serving, Calories: 233- Fat: 14.7g - Carbs: 8.7g - Protein: 18.6g

Ingredients:

- 2 tbsp. of extra-virgin olive oil

- 1½ pound of lean ground turkey

- 2 chopped medium onions

- 1 chopped large celery stalk

- 4 minced garlic cloves

- 1 seeded and chopped jalapeño pepper

- 1 tsp. of crushed dried oregano

- 2 cups of chopped tomatoes

- 1 cup of small cauliflower florets

- 1 cup of small broccoli florets

- 7 cups of water

- 1 peeled, pitted and chopped avocado

- Sea salt and freshly ground black pepper, to taste

Directions:

1. In a medium pan, heat oil on medium-high.

2. Add turkey and cook for about 8-10 minutes or till browned completely.

3. Add onion, celery and garlic and sauté for about 5 minutes.

4. Add jalapeño pepper, oregano and tomatoes and cook for about 2-3 minutes, crushing with the back of the spoon.

5. Add the cauliflower and broccoli and cook for about 3-4 minutes.

6. Add water, salt and pepper and bring to a boil.

7. Reduce the heat to low and simmer, covered for about 30-40 minutes or till desired doneness.

8. Stir in avocado and simmer for about 5 minutes.

9. Serve hot.

Protein-Rich Stew (6 servings, serving: 1 bowl)

Per Serving, Calories: 238- Fat: 3.9g - Carbs: 39.9g - Protein: 12.4g

Ingredients:

- 1 tbsp. of olive oil

- 3 chopped celery stalks

- 3 peeled and chopped carrots

- 1 chopped onion

- 2 minced garlic cloves

- 1 cup of rinsed and drained red lentils

- ½ cup of rinsed and drained quinoa

- 3 cups of chopped tomatoes

- 1½ tsp. of ground cumin

- ½ tsp. of ground ginger

- ½ tsp. of ground turmeric

- Sea salt and freshly ground black pepper, to taste

- 5 cups of water

- 2 cups of trimmed and chopped fresh kale

Directions:

1. In a large pan, heat oil on medium heat.

2. Add celery, carrot and onion and sauté for about 8 minutes.

3. Add garlic and spices and sauté for about 1 minute.

4. Stir in remaining ingredients except kale and bring to a boil.

5. Reduce the heat to low and simmer, covered for about 20 minutes.

6. Stir in kale and simmer for about 4-5 minutes.

7. Serve hot.

Creamy Chickpeas Stew (8 servings, serving: 1 bowl)

Per Serving, Calories: 399- Fat: 14.9g - Carbs: 54.4g - Protein: 16.1g

Ingredients:

- 2 tbsp. of olive oil

- 1 chopped medium yellow onion

- 2 tsp. of finely chopped fresh ginger

- 2 minced garlic cloves

- 1 tsp. of ground cumin

- 1 tsp. of ground coriander

- ¾ tsp. of ground turmeric

- ¼ tsp. of cayenne pepper

- 1 (19-ounce) can of rinsed and drained low-sodium chickpeas

- 1 peeled and cubed into 1-inch size large sweet potatoes

- 1 pound of trimmed and chopped fresh kale

- 5 cups of water

- 1 cup of unsweetened coconut milk

- ¼ cup of chopped fresh cilantro

Directions:

1. In a large pan, heat oil on medium heat.

2. Add onion and sauté for about 3 minutes.

3. Add ginger and garlic and sauté for about 2 minutes.

4. Add spices and sauté for about 1 minute.

5. Add chickpeas, sweet potato, kale and broth and bring to a boil on medium-high heat.

6. Reduce the heat to medium-low and simmer, covered for about 35 minutes.

7. Stir in coconut milk and simmer for about 15 minutes or till desired thickness of stew.

8. Serve hot with garnishing of bell pepper and cilantro.

Scrumptious Stew (6 servings, serving: 1 bowl)

Per Serving, Calories: 112- Fat: 4.8g - Carbs: 10.4g - Protein: 10.3g

Ingredients:

- 1 (16-ounce) jar of rinsed and drained roasted red peppers

- 1 seeded and chopped jalapeño pepper

- 2¼ cups of fat-free, low-sodium vegetable broth, divided

- 2 cups of water

- 1 seeded and thinly sliced medium red bell pepper

- 1 seeded and thinly sliced medium green bell pepper

- 1 (16-ounce) package of drained and cubed extra-firm tofu

- 1 (10-ounce) package of thawed frozen baby spinach

Directions:

1. In a food processor, add roasted red peppers, jalapeño pepper and ¼ cup of broth and pulse till a smooth puree forms.

2. In a large pan, mix together puree, broth and water on medium-high heat and bring to a boil.

3. Stir in bell peppers and tofu and again bring to a boil.

4. Reduce the heat to medium and cook for about 5 minutes.

5. Stir in spinach and cook for about 5 minutes.

6. Serve hot.

Great Entrée Stew (4 servings, serving: 1 bowl)

Per Serving, Calories: 284- Fat: 13.5g - Carbs: 13.6g - Protein: 27.2g

Ingredients:

- 2 tbsp. of olive oil, divided

- 3 (4-ounce) grass-fed skinless, boneless chicken breasts

- Pinch of sea salt

- Freshly ground black pepper, to taste

- 1 chopped medium yellow onion

- 2 minced garlic cloves

- ¾ cup of homemade tomato puree, divided

- 3 cups of fat-free, low-sodium chicken broth

- 2 peeled and chopped small sweet potatoes

- ½ cup of chopped fresh cilantro

Directions:

1. In a large pan, heat 1 tbsp. of oil on medium heat.

2. Add chicken and sprinkle with salt and black pepper and cook for about 4-5 minutes per side.

3. Transfer the chicken in a large bowl and keep aside.

4. In the same pan, heat remaining oil on medium heat.

5. Add onion and sauté for about 3-4 minutes.

6. Add garlic, dried herbs, spices, and 1 tbsp. of tomato puree and sauté for about 1 minute.

7. Add chicken, remaining tomato puree and broth and bring to a boil.

8. Reduce the heat to low and simmer, covered for about 1½ hours.

9. Remove chicken from pan and keep aside to cool slightly.

10. Cut chicken into desired pieces.

11. Add sweet potato and chicken pieces in pan and bring to a boil on medium heat.

12. Reduce the heat to low and simmer, covered for about 30 minutes.

13. Stir in spinach and black pepper and simmer for about 5 minutes.

14. Serve hot with the garnishing of cilantro.

Omega-3 Rich Stew (6 servings, serving: 1 bowl)

Per Serving, Calories: 224- Fat: 12g - Carbs: 6.7g - Protein: 24.2g

Ingredients:

- 2 tbsp. of olive oil

- ½ cup of finely chopped onion

- 2 minced garlic cloves

- 1 chopped Serrano pepper

- 1 tsp. of smoked paprika

- 4 cups of chopped fresh tomatoes

- 4 cups of fat-free, low-sodium chicken broth

- 1½ pound of cubed boneless salmon fillets

- 2 tbsp. of fresh lime juice

- 3 tbsp. of chopped fresh basil

- 3 tbsp. of chopped fresh parsley

- Freshly ground black pepper, to taste

- 2 chopped scallions

Directions:

1. In a large soup pan, melt coconut oil on medium-high heat.

2. Add onion and sauté for about 5-6 minutes.

3. Add garlic, Serrano pepper and smoked paprika and sauté for about 1 minute.

4. Add tomatoes and broth and bring to a gentle simmer on medium heat.

5. Simmer for about 5 minutes.

6. Add salmon and simmer for about 6-8 minutes.

7. Stir in lemon juice, basil, parsley and black pepper and remove from heat.

8. Serve hot with the garnishing of scallion.

Weeknight Dinner Chili (10 servings, serving: 1 bowl)

Per Serving, Calories: 462- Fat: 5.3g - Carbs: 80.2g - Protein: 27.1g

Ingredients:

- 2 tbsp. of canola oil

- 2 chopped medium onions

- 5 minced garlic cloves

- 2 seeded and chopped jalapeño peppers

- ¾ tbsp. of crushed dried basil

- ¾ tbsp. of crushed dried oregano

- 3 tbsp. of red chili powder

- 2 tbsp. of ground cumin

- 2 tbsp. of ground coriander

- 1 tsp. of ground cinnamon

- ¼ cup of homemade tomato puree

- 4¼ cups of fat-free, low sodium vegetable broth

- 6 cups of cooked black beans

- 3 cups of chopped tomatoes

- Freshly ground black pepper, to taste

- ½ cup of chopped fresh cilantro

Directions:

1. In a large pan, heat oil on medium-high heat.

2. Add onion and sauté for about 8-9 minutes.

3. Add garlic, jalapeño peppers, herbs and spices and sauté for about 1 minute.

4. Add tomato puree, broth, black beans and tomatoes and bring to a boil.

5. Reduce the heat to low and simmer, covered for about 1 hour.

6. Season with black pepper and remove from heat.

7. Serve hot with the garnishing of cilantro.

Richly Tasty Chili (8 servings, serving: 1 bowl)

Per Serving, Calories: 253- Fat: 2.9g - Carbs: 41g - Protein: 16.5g

Ingredients:

- 3 tsp. of canola oil

- 1 chopped large onion

- 3 peeled and chopped medium carrots

- 4 chopped celery stalks

- 2 minced garlic cloves

- 1 seeded and chopped jalapeño pepper

- 2 tbsp. of tomato paste

- 1 tbsp. of chipotle chili powder

- 1½ tbsp. of ground coriander

- 1½ tbsp. of ground cumin

- 1½ tsp. of ground turmeric

- Freshly ground black pepper, to taste

- 1 pound of rinsed lentils

- 6 cups of fat-free, low sodium vegetable broth

- ¼ cup of chopped fresh mint leaves

- ¼ cup of chopped fresh cilantro

Directions:

1. In a large pan, heat oil on medium heat.

2. Add onion, carrot and celery and sauté for about 5 minutes.

3. Add garlic, jalapeño pepper and spices and sauté for about 1 minute.

4. Add tomato paste, lentils and broth and bring to a boil.

5. Reduce the heat to low and simmer for about 2 hours.

6. Stir in spinach and simmer for about 3-4 minutes.

7. Serve hot with the garnishing of mint and cilantro.

Stunning Dinner Curry (4 servings, serving: 1 bowl)

Per Serving, Calories: 266- Fat: 10g - Carbs: 41g - Protein: 9.9g

Ingredients:

- 2 tbsp. of olive oil

- 2 chopped onion

- 4 minced garlic cloves

- 3 tbsp. of curry powder

- Freshly ground black pepper, to taste

- 2/3 cup of fat-free plain Greek yogurt

- 1 cup of homemade tomato paste

- 2 peeled and sliced bananas

- 3 chopped fresh tomatoes

- ¼ cup of unsweetened coconut flakes

Directions:

1. In a large pan, heat oil on medium heat.

2. Add onion and sauté for about 4-5 minutes.

3. Add garlic, curry powder, sugar and spices and sauté for about 1 minute.

4. Add yogurt and tomato sauce and bring to a gentle boil.

5. Stir in bananas and simmer for about 3 minutes.

6. Stir in tomatoes and simmer for about 1-2 minutes.

7. Stir in coconut flakes and immediately remove from heat.

8. Serve hot.

Satisfying Curry (4 servings, serving: 1 bowl)

Per Serving, Calories: 394- Fat: 8.3g - Carbs: 61.3g - Protein: 8.7 g

Ingredients:

- 2 tbsp. of olive oil

- 1 finely chopped medium onion

- ½ tbsp. of finely grated fresh ginger

- 2 minced garlic cloves

- 1 seeded and chopped green chili

- ½ tbsp. of ground cumin

- ½ tbsp. of ground coriander

- ¼ tsp. of ground turmeric

- ½ cup of finely chopped tomatoes

- 2 cups of cooked red kidney beans

- ½ cup of fat-free, low sodium vegetable broth

- Freshly ground black pepper, to taste

- 2 tbsp. of chopped fresh cilantro

Directions:

1. In a large pan, heat oil on medium heat.

2. Add onion and sauté for 6-8 minutes.

3. Add ginger, garlic, green chili and spices and sauté for about 1 minute.

4. Add tomatoes and cook for about 5-6 minutes, crushing with the back of spoon.

5. Add kidney beans and broth and bring to a boil on medium-high heat.

6. Reduce the heat to medium-low and simmer for about 4-5 minutes or till desired consistency.

7. Season with black pepper and remove from heat.

8. Garnish with cilantro and serve.

Lively Flavored Curry (4 servings, serving: 1 bowl)

Per Serving, Calories: 221- Fat: 4.3g - Carbs: 33.1g - Protein: 13.3g

Ingredients:

For Tomato Puree:

- 1 cup of chopped tomatoes

- 1 chopped garlic clove

- 1 chopped green chili

- ¼ cup of water

For Lentils:

- 3 cups of water

- 1 cup of red lentils

- 1 tbsp. of canola oil

- ½ of chopped medium onion

- ½ tsp. of ground cumin

- ½ tsp. of cayenne pepper

- ¼ tsp. of ground turmeric

- ¼ cup of chopped tomato

- ¼ cup of chopped fresh parsley leaves

Directions:

1. For tomato paste in a blender, add all ingredients and pulse till a smooth puree forms. Keep aside.

2. In a large pan, add 3 cups of water and lentils on high heat and bring to a boil.

3. Reduce the heat to medium-low and simmer, covered for about 15-20 minutes or till tender enough. Drain the lentils.

4. In a large skillet, heat oil on medium heat.

5. Add onion and sauté for about 6-7 minutes.

6. Add spices and sauté for about 1 minute.

7. Add tomato puree and cook for about 5-7 minutes, stirring occasionally.

8. Stir in lentils and cook for about 4-5 minutes or till desired doneness.

9. Stir in chopped tomato and immediately remove from heat.

10. Serve hot with the garnishing of parsley.

Green Chicken Curry (5 servings, serving: 1 bowl)

Per Serving, Calories: 259- Fat: 19.1g - Carbs: 7.3g - Protein: 16.2g

Ingredients:

- 1 tbsp. of olive oil

- 2 tbsp. of green curry paste

- 2 cubed grass-fed skinless, boneless chicken breasts

- 1 cup of unsweetened coconut milk

- 1 cup of fat-free, low-sodium chicken broth

- 1 cup of trimmed asparagus spears

- 1 cup of trimmed green beans

- Freshly ground black pepper, to taste

- ¼ cup of chopped fresh cilantro leaves

Directions:

In a skillet, heat oil on medium heat.

Add green curry paste and sauté for about 1-2 minutes.

Add chicken and cook for about 8-10 minutes.

Add coconut milk and broth and bring to a boil.

Reduce the heat low and simmer for about 8-10 minutes.

Add asparagus, green beans and black pepper and cook for about 4-5 minutes or till desired doneness.

Serve with the garnishing of cilantro.

Holiday Favorite Gratin (6 servings, serving: 1 portion)

Per Serving, Calories: 377- Fat: 19.9g - Carbs: 49g - Protein: 4.4g

Ingredients:

- 2 tbsp. of olive oil

- ¼ cup of almond flour

- 1½ cups of unsweetened coconut milk

- 1 minced garlic clove

- 1 tsp. of crushed dried thyme

- Sea salt, to taste

- 2/3 cup of homemade pumpkin puree

- 2 pound of peeled and cut into 1/8-inch thick slices sweet potatoes

- 1 thinly sliced shallot

Directions:

1. Preheat the oven to 400 degrees F. Grease an 11x7-inch baking dish.

2. In a pan, melt coconut butter on medium heat

3. Slowly, add flour, stirring continuously till a crumbly mixture forms.

4. Slowly, add milk, stirring continuously till well combined.

5. Stir in thyme, garlic powder and salt.

6. Stir in pumpkin puree till well combined and smooth.

7. Meanwhile divide sweet potato slices in 4 portions.

8. Divide shallot in 3 portions.

9. Arrange 1 portion of sweet potato slices in the bottom of prepared baking dish.

10. Place 1 portion of shallot over sweet potato slices. Repeat with the layers, topping with last portion of sweet potato.

11. Place pumpkin mixture over sweet potato slices evenly.

12. Bake for about 30-40 minutes or till top becomes golden brown.

Flavorsome Vegan Dinner (5 servings, serving: 1 portion)

Per Serving, Calories: 470- Fat: 13.6g - Carbs: 72.6g - Protein: 18.7g

Ingredients:

For Vegetables:

- 2 halved large sweet potatoes

- ½ of sliced in wedges red onion

- 2 tbsp. of olive oil, divided

- ½ pound of stemmed and chopped broccolini,

- 2 cups of trimmed fresh kale

- Sea salt and freshly ground black pepper, to taste

For Chickpeas:

- 1 tbsp. of olive oil

- 2 cups of cooked chickpeas

- ¼ tsp. of finely grated fresh ginger

- ½ tsp. of crushed dried oregano

- ½ tsp. of red chili powder

- ¼ tsp. of crushed red pepper flakes

- ¼ tsp. of ground cumin

- ¼ tsp. of ground turmeric

Directions:

1. Preheat the oven to 400 degrees F.

2. Drizzle sweet potato halves and onion with 1 tbsp. of oil.

3. Place sweet potato in a baking sheet, cut side up.

4. Arrange onion wedges around sweet potato.

5. Bake for about 10 minutes.

6. Remove the baking sheet from oven. Change the side of sweet potato halves.

7. Meanwhile in a bowl, add broccolini, ½ tbsp. of oil and a pinch of salt and black pepper and toss to coat well.

8. Transfer the broccolini in baking sheet. Bake for about 10 minutes.

9. Meanwhile in a bowl, add kale, remaining oil and a pinch of Sea salt and black pepper and toss to coat well.

10. Transfer the kale in baking sheet.

11. Bake for about 4-5 minutes. Remove from oven.

12. Then peel and cut the sweet potato in desired sized slices.

13. Meanwhile in a skillet, heat oil on medium heat.

14. Add ginger and sauté for about 30 seconds.

15. Add chickpeas and remaining all ingredients and sauté for about 8-10 minutes.

16. Divide the vegetable mixture in serving plates.

17. Top with chickpeas and serve.

Meat-Less Loaf (8 servings, serving: 1 portion)

Per Serving, Calories: 190- Fat: 5.5g - Carbs: 28.9g - Protein: 9.6g

Ingredients:

- 1¾ cups plus 2 tbsp. of water, divided

- ½ cup of wild rice

- ½ cup of brown lentils

- Sea salt, to taste

- 1 chopped medium yellow onion

- 1 chopped celery stalk

- 6 chopped cremini mushrooms

- 4 minced garlic cloves

- ¾ cup of rolled oats

- ½ cup of finely chopped walnuts

- ¾ cup of sugar-free, low-sodium ketchup

- ½ tsp. of crushed red pepper flakes

- 1 tsp. of minced fresh rosemary

- 2 tsp. of minced fresh thyme

Directions:

1. In a pan, add 1¾ cups f water, rice, lentils and salt on medium-high heat and bring to a boil.

2. Reduce the heat to low and simmer, covered for about 45 minutes.

3. Remove from heat and keep aside, covered for at least 10 minutes.

4. Preheat the oven to 350 degrees F. Line 9x5-inch loaf pan with parchment paper.

5. In a skillet, heat remaining water on medium heat.

6. Add onion, celery, mushrooms, garlic and sauté for about 4-5 minutes.

7. Remove from heat and keep aside to cool slightly.

8. In a large bowl, add oats, walnuts, ketchup and fresh herbs and mix till well combined.

9. Add rice mixture and vegetable mixture and mix well.

10. In a blender add mixture and pulse till just a chunky mixture forms.

11. Transfer the mixture into prepared loaf pan evenly.

12. With a piece of the foil, cover the loaf and bake for about 40 minutes.

13. Uncover and bake for about 15-20 minutes more or till top becomes golden brown.

Entertaining Casserole (6 servings, serving: 1 portion)

Per Serving, Calories: 372- Fat: 10.8g - Carbs: 58g - Protein: 13.8g

Ingredients:

For Sauce:

- 1 cup of shelled, soaked for 30 minutes, drained and rinsed sunflower seeds

- ¼ cup of low-sodium tamari

- Pinch of crushed red pepper flakes, crushed

- 1½ cups of water

For Casserole:

- 1 (14-ounce) package of whole wheat fusilli pasta

- 2 tbsp. of canola oil

- 1 minced garlic clove

- 2 chopped Serrano peppers

- ¼ tsp. of ground cumin

- 3 cups of trimmed and cut into 4 sections fresh Brussels sprouts

- Freshly ground black pepper, to taste

- 1 cup of water

- 1 (14-ounce) package of thawed frozen spinach

Directions:

1. Preheat the oven to 400 degrees F. Grease large baking dish.

2. For sauce in a blender, add all ingredients and pulse till smooth.

3. Transfer into a bowl and keep aside.

4. In a pan of Sea salted boiling water, add pasta and cook for about 8-10 minutes.

5. Drain well and keep aside.

6. Meanwhile in a large skillet, heat oil on medium heat.

7. Add garlic, Serrano peppers and cumin and sauté for about 1 minute.

8. Add Brussels sprouts, Sea salt and black pepper and cook for about 3-4 minutes.

9. Add water and cook for about 8-10 minutes.

10. Stir in spinach and cook for about 1 minute.

11. Stir in sunflower sauce and cook for about 1 minute.

12. Stir in cooked pasta and hot sauce and remove from heat.

13. Transfer the pasta mixture into prepared baking dish.

14. Bake for about 35 minutes.

Decadent Casserole (5 servings, serving: 1 portion)

Per Serving, Calories: 311- Fat: 18.7g - Carbs: 22.8g - Protein: 18.7g

Ingredients:

- 3 tbsp. of canola oil, divided

- 2 (8-ounce) packages of cut into ½-inch slices horizontally tempeh

- 1 chopped large onion

- 3 minced garlic cloves

- 1 tsp. of crushed dried oregano

- 1 tsp. of crushed dried thyme

- 1 tsp. of paprika

- ½ tsp. of crushed red pepper flakes

- 2 seeded and thinly sliced large green bell peppers

- 2 cups of finely chopped tomatoes

- ¼ cup of homemade tomato puree

- 1 tsp. of balsamic vinegar

- 1 tbsp. of maple syrup

Directions:

1. Preheat the oven to 350 degrees F.

2. In a large nonstick skillet, heat 2 tbsp. of oil on medium-high heat.

3. Add tempeh slices and cook for about 5-7 minutes.

4. Carefully, change the side and cook for about 5-7 minutes.

5. Transfer the cooked tempeh slices into a paper towel lined plate. Keep aside.

6. Meanwhile in another nonstick skillet, heat remaining oil on medium-low heat.

7. Add onion, garlic, herbs and spices and sauté for about 8-10 minutes.

8. Add bell pepper and sauté for about 10 minutes.

9. Add remaining ingredients and stir till well combined.

10. Transfer the tempeh slices in a large casserole dish.

11. Place tomato mixture over tempeh slices evenly.

12. With a piece of foil, cover the casserole dish.

13. Bake for about 1 hour.

Party Dinner Casserole (3 servings, serving: 1 portion)

Per Serving, Calories: 206- Fat: 5g - Carbs: 35g - Protein: 6.1g

Ingredients:

- 1 tsp. of extra-virgin olive oil

- 1 thinly sliced red onion

- 1½ tsp. of ground turmeric

- 9-ounce of sliced brown mushrooms

- 1 tsp. of raisins

- ½ cup of rinsed brown rice

- 1¼ cups of fat-free, low sodium vegetable broth

- ¼ cup of chopped fresh cilantro

- 1 tbsp. of toasted pine nuts

- 1 tbsp. of fresh lemon juice

- Freshly ground black pepper, to taste

Directions:

1. Preheat the oven to 400 degrees F.

2. In an ovenproof casserole, heat oil on medium heat and sauté onion and turmeric for about 3 minutes.

3. Add mushrooms and stir fry for about 2 minutes.

4. Stir in raisins, rice and broth and immediately, transfer into oven.

5. Bake for about 45-55 minutes or until desired doneness.

6. Stir in remaining ingredients and serve immediately.

Enticing Casserole (6 servings, serving: 1 portion)

Per Serving, Calories: 190- Fat: 7.6g - Carbs: 23.3g - Protein: 12.7g

Ingredients:

- 1 tbsp. of olive oil

- 1 chopped yellow onion

- 3 mined cloves garlic, minced

- 1 tbsp. of minced fresh ginger

- 4 cups of thinly sliced cabbage

- 4 peeled and sliced carrots

- 1 sliced fennel bulb

- ½ pound of snap peas

- ½ tbsp. of ground coriander

- ½ tbsp. of ground cumin

- 1½ tsp. of ground turmeric

- Pinch of cayenne pepper

- 8-ounce of cut into small chunks tempeh

- 2 cups of fat-free low-sodium vegetable broth

Directions:

1. In a skillet, heat oil on medium heat.

2. Add onion, garlic and ginger, and garlic and sauté for about 5 minutes.

3. Add cabbage, carrots, fennel, and snap peas and sauté for about 3 minutes.

4. Stir in spices and tempeh chunks and broth and bring to a boil.

5. Reduce the heat to low and simmer, covered for about10-15 minutes.

6. Serve hot.

Flavorsome Chicken (4 servings, serving: 1 portion)

Per Serving, Calories: 277- Fat: 4.2g - Carbs: 17.9g - Protein: 21.4g

Ingredients:

- 2 tbsp. of olive oil

- 1 chopped medium onion

- 1 seeded and chopped medium green bell pepper

- 1 minced garlic clove

- ½ tsp. of minced fresh ginger

- 2 (6-ounce) cut into 1-inch pieces grass-fed skinless, boneless chicken breasts

- ¼ cup of raw cashews

- 2 tbsp. honey

- 1 tbsp. of balsamic vinegar

- 1 tbsp. of low-sodium tamari

- 3 chopped scallions

- Freshly ground black pepper, to taste

Directions:

1. In a large skillet, heat oil on medium heat.

2. Add onion and bell pepper and sauté for about 4-5 minutes.

3. Add garlic and ginger and sauté for about 1 minute.

4. Add chicken and cook for about 4-5 minutes.

5. Stir in cashews and cook for about 3-4 minutes.

6. Stir in honey, vinegar and tamari and cook for about 4-5 minutes.

7. Stir in scallion and black pepper and immediately remove from heat.

8. Serve hot.

Deliciously Spicy Chicken (6 servings, serving: 1 portion)

Per Serving, Calories: 275- Fat: 17.8g - Carbs: 6.4g - Protein: 23.5g

Ingredients:

For Spice Mixture:

- 1 tsp. of ground coriander

- 1 tsp. of ground cumin

- ¼ tsp. of ground cinnamon

- 1 tsp. of crushed red pepper flakes

- ¼ tsp. of red chili powder

- ¼ tsp. of ground turmeric

- 1 bay leaf

- Sea salt, to taste

For Coconut Mixture:

- ¼ cup of grated coconut

- ½ tbsp. of peeled fresh ginger

- 3 chopped garlic cloves

- 1 chopped fresh green chili

- ¼ cup of water

For Chicken:

- 2 tbsp. of olive oil

- 1 chopped large white onion

- 1 pound of cubed grass-fed skinless boneless chicken breasts

- 1 cup of unsweetened coconut milk

- ¼ cup of chopped fresh cilantro

Directions:

1. For spice blend in a small bowl, mix together all spices. Keep aside.

2. For coconut mixture in a blender, add all ingredients and pulse till a smooth paste forms.

3. Transfer the paste into a bowl. Keep aside.

4. In a large skillet, heat 1 tbsp. of of oil on medium-high heat.

5. Add chicken and cook, stirring occasionally for about 4-5 minutes or till browned from all sides.

6. Transfer the chicken into a bowl.

7. In the same skillet, heat remaining oil on medium heat.

8. Add onion and sauté for about 4-5 minutes.

9. Stir in spice blend and sauté for about 1 minute.

10. Stir in coconut mixture and sauté for about 3-4minutes.

11. Stir in cooked chicken and cook for about 1 minute.

12. Add coconut milk and bring to a boil.

13. Reduce the heat to low and simmer, covered for about 20-25 minutes or till desired thickness of gravy.

14. Serve hot with the garnishing of cilantro.

Strengthening Dinner Meal (6 servings, serving: 1 portion)

Per Serving, Calories: 357- Fat: 25.3g - Carbs: 9.8g - Protein: 25.7g

Ingredients:

- 13-ounce of unsweetened coconut milk
- 1 tsp. of grated fresh ginger
- 1½ tsp. of curry powder
- 2 tbsp. of olive oil, divided
- 1 pound of thinly sliced grass-fed skinless, boneless chicken breasts
- 1 chopped large onion
- 2 cups of broccoli florets
- 1 large bunch of chopped fresh spinach

Directions:

1. In a bowl, mix together coconut milk, ginger and curry powder. Keep aside.
2. In a large skillet, heat 1 tbsp. of oil on medium-high heat.
3. Add chicken and stir fry for about 4-5 minutes or till golden brown completely.
4. Transfer chicken into a plate.
5. In the same skillet, heat remaining oil on medium-high heat.
6. Add onion and sauté for about 2 minutes.
7. Add broccoli and stir fry for about 3 minutes.
8. Add chicken, spinach and coconut mixture and stir fry for about 3-4 minutes.

9. Serve hot.

Delish Chicken Platter (6 servings, serving: 1 portion)

Per Serving, Calories: 230- Fat: 9.5g - Carbs: 18.3g - Protein: 20.1g

Ingredients:

- 2 tbsp. of extra-virgin olive oil

- 2 (6-ounce) sliced grass-fed skinless, boneless chicken breasts

- 1 thinly sliced red onion

- 2 minced garlic cloves

- 2 tbsp. of minced fresh ginger

- 1 ripe, peeled, pitted and cubed mango

- 2 cups of chopped broccoli

- 1 cup of sliced zucchini

- 1 cup of sliced mushrooms, sliced

- 1 seeded and cubed red bell pepper

- 3 tbsp. of low-sodium tamari

- ¼ tsp. of crushed red chili flakes

- Freshly ground black pepper, to taste

- ¼ cup of sliced scallion

Directions:

1. In a large skillet, heat oil on medium-high heat.

2. Add chicken and stir fry for about 4-5 minutes or till golden brown.

3. Transfer chicken into a plate.

4. In the same skillet, add onion, garlic and ginger and sauté for about 1-2 minutes.

5. Add mango, broccoli, zucchini and bell pepper and cook for about 5-7 minutes.

6. Add chicken, tamari, red chili flakes and black pepper and cook for about 3-4 minutes or till desired doneness.

7. Serve with the topping of scallion.

Family Feast Dinner (5 servings, serving: 1 portion)

Per Serving, Calories: 242- Fat: 7.8g - Carbs: 11.2g - Protein: 29.7g

Ingredients:

- 1 pound of grass-fed lean ground beef

- 1 tbsp. of olive oil

- 1 chopped small onion

- 1 minced garlic clove

- 1 seeded and chopped small red bell pepper

- 1 seeded and chopped small yellow bell pepper

- 1 seeded and chopped small green bell pepper

- 3 cups of trimmed and chopped fresh kale

- Sea salt and freshly ground black pepper, to taste

- 1 tbsp. of fresh lemon juice

Directions:

1. Heat a large skillet on medium-high heat.

2. Add the beef and cook for about 8-10 minutes or till browned completely.

3. Transfer the beef into a bowl and drain the grease from the skillet.

4. In the same skillet, heat the oil on medium heat.

5. Add onion and garlic and sauté for about 4-5 minutes.

6. Add bell peppers and cook for about 4-5 minutes.

7. Add beef and kale cook for about 4-5 minutes.

8. Stir in salt, black pepper and lemon juice and serve immediately.

Succulent Lamb Chops (8 servings, serving: 1 portion)

Per Serving, Calories: 384- Fat: 15.8g - Carbs: 29g - Protein: 33g

Ingredients:

For Lamb Chops:

- 2 tbsp. of olive oil

- 2 minced garlic cloves

- ½ tbsp. of finely chopped fresh rosemary

- ½ tbsp. of finely chopped fresh thyme

- ½ tsp. of ground cumin

- ¼ tsp. of ground turmeric

- ¼ tsp. of crushed red pepper flakes

- 8 (4-ounce) trimmed grass-fed lamb rib chops

- Pinch of sea salt

- Freshly ground black pepper, to taste

For Onion & Apple:

- 2 tbsp. of olive oil

- 6 cored and sliced medium apples

- 3 sliced large red onions

- Sea salt and freshly ground black pepper, to taste

Directions:

1. In a large skillet, heat oil on medium heat.

2. Add garlic, rosemary, thyme, cumin and red pepper flakes and sauté for about 1 minute.

3. Add lamb chops and sprinkle with Sea salt and black pepper.

4. Cook for about 3-4 minutes per side or till desired doneness.

5. Meanwhile in another skillet, heat oil on medium-low heat.

6. Add inions and apples and sprinkle with a little salt and black pepper.

7. Cook for about 4-5 minutes. Remove from heat and divide apple mixture into 4 portions.

8. Place 1 lamb chop in each serving plate and top with the apple mixture evenly.

9. Serve immediately.

Exceptionally Tasty Salmon (6 servings, serving: 1 portion)

Per Serving, Calories: 181- Fat: 7.2g - Carbs: 6.1g - Protein: 24.7g

Ingredients:

- 1½ pound of asparagus spears

- 1/3 cup of fresh orange juice

- 2 tbsp. of fresh lemon juice

- 1 cup of water

- 6 (4-ounce) skinless, boneless salmon fillets

- 3 tbsp. of chopped parsley

- Sea salt and freshly ground black pepper, to taste

Directions:

1. In a pan of boiling water, cook the asparagus for about 2-3 minutes.

2. Drain well.

3. In a large skillet, add orange juice, lemon juice and water and bring to boil on high heat.

4. Stir in the salmon fillets and cook on medium heat for about 6-7 minutes.

5. Add the asparagus, parsley, salt and black pepper and cook for about 2-3 minutes.

6. Serve hot.

Family Dinner Salmon (2 servings, serving: 1 portion)

Per Serving, Calories: 299- Fat: 21.3g - Carbs: 5.6g - Protein: 24g

Ingredients:

- 2 tbsp. of olive oil, divided

- 2 minced garlic cloves

- 2 tsp. of finely grated fresh ginger

- 2 (4-ounce) salmon fillet

- Pinch of sea salt

- Freshly ground black pepper, to taste

- 1 finely chopped Serrano pepper

- 4 cups of roughly chopped Swiss chard

- 2 tsp. of low-sodium tamari

Directions:

1. In a skillet, heat 1 tbsp. of oil on medium heat.

2. Add garlic and ginger and sauté for about 1 minute.

3. Add salmon fillet and sprinkle with salt and black pepper.

4. Cook for about 4-5 minutes per side or till desired doneness.

5. Meanwhile in another skillet, heat remaining oil on medium heat.

6. Add Serrano pepper and sauté for about 30 seconds.

7. Add Swiss chard and tamari and cook for about 5-10 minutes.

8. Serve the salmon fillet over Swiss chard.

CHAPTER 4: SNACK RECIPES

Appealing Party Treat (4 servings, serving: 1 portion)

Per Serving, Calories: 179- Fat: 17g - Carbs: 7.9g - Protein: 1.7g

Ingredients:

- 1 cut in 1-inch thick slices large cucumber

- 1 peeled and finely chopped ripe avocado,

- ½ of peeled, seeded and finely chopped medium tomato

- 2 tbsp. of fresh lemon juice

- 2 tbsp. of olive oil

- ¼ tsp. of cayenne pepper

- Sea salt, to taste

Directions:

1. Scoop out the inside of each cucumber slice, leaving the bottom intact so it resembles a cup.

2. In a blender, add remaining ingredients and pulse till smooth and creamy.

3. Spoon the avocado mixture into each cucumber cup.

4. Serve immediately.

Chunky Tomato Relish (3 servings, serving: 1 portion)

Per Serving, Calories: 79- Fat: 0.5g - Carbs: 18.5g - Protein: 2.6g

Ingredients:

- 2 tsp. of arrowroot starch

- 1 tbsp. of water

- 3 cups of seeded and chopped frozen bell peppers

- ¾ cup of chopped tomato

- 2/3 cup of frozen onions

- ½ cup of tomato puree

- 1 tbsp. of cider vinegar

- Sea salt, to taste

Directions:

1. In a small bowl, mix together cornstarch and water.

2. In a pan, mix together arrowroot starch mixture and remaining ingredients on medium-low heat.

3. Simmer for about 3-5 minutes, , stirring continuously.

4. Transfer the relish in a bowl and refrigerate before serving.

Naturally Sweet Guacamole (8 servings, serving: 1 portion)

Per Serving, Calories: 137- Fat: 10g - Carbs: 12.8g - Protein: 1.5g

Ingredients:

- 2 peeled, pitted and roughly chopped large ripe avocados

- 1 cup of hulled and chopped fresh strawberries

- 1 cup of peeled, pitted and chopped mango

- 1 chopped small red onion

- 1 tbsp. of fresh lime juice

- ¼ cup of chopped fresh cilantro leaves

Directions:

1. In a large serving bowl, add all ingredients and gently stir to combine.

2. Serve immediately.

Kids Friendly Fries (3 servings, serving: 1 portion)

Per Serving, Calories: 90- Fat: 4.8g - Carbs: 11.4g - Protein: 1.1g

Ingredients:

- 1 peeled and cut into wedges large sweet potato

- 1 tsp. of ground turmeric

- 1 tsp. of ground cinnamon

- Sea salt and freshly ground black pepper, to taste

- 1 tbsp. of extra-virgin olive oil

Directions:

1. Preheat the oven to 425 degrees F. Line a baking sheet with a foil paper.

2. In a large bowl, add all ingredients and toss to coat well.

3. Transfer the mixture into prepared baking sheet.

4. Bake for about 25 minutes, flipping once after 15 minutes.

5. Serve immediately.

Unique Pumpkin Seeds (6 servings, serving: 1 portion)

Per Serving, Calories: 185- Fat: 17.6g - Carbs: 4.3g - Protein: 5.7g

Ingredients:

- 1 cup of washed and dried pumpkin seeds

- 1/3 tsp. of red chili powder

- ¼ tsp. of ground turmeric

- Pinch of sea salt

- 3 tbsp. of olive oil

- ½ tbsp. of fresh lemon juice

Directions:

1. Preheat the oven to 350 degrees F.

2. In a bowl, add all ingredients except lemon juice and toss to coat well.

3. Transfer the almond mixture into a baking sheet.

4. Roast for about 20 minutes, flipping occasionally.

5. Remove from oven and keep aside to cool completely before serving.

6. Drizzle with lemon juice and serve.

Welcoming Roasted Cashews (16 servings, serving: 1 portion)

Per Serving, Calories: 106- Fat: 8.3g - Carbs: 6.8g - Protein: 2.7g

Ingredients:

- 2 cups of cashews

- 2 tsp. of honey

- 1½ tsp. of smoked paprika

- ½ tsp. of chili flakes

- Pinch of sea salt

- 1 tbsp. of fresh lemon juice

- 1 tsp. of olive oil

Directions:

1. Preheat the oven to 350 degrees F. Line a baking dish with the parchment paper.

2. In a bowl, add all ingredients and toss to coat well.

3. Transfer the cashew mixture into prepared baking dish in a single layer.

4. Roast for about 20 minutes, flipping once in the middle way.

5. Remove from oven and keep aside to cool completely before serving.

6. You can preserve these roasted cashews in airtight jar.

Loveable Apple Leather (6 servings, serving: 1 portion)

Per Serving, Calories: 159- Fat: 0.6g - Carbs: 42.1g - Protein: 0.9g

Ingredients:

- 1 cup of water

- 8 cups of peeled, cored and chopped apples

- 1 tbsp. of ground cinnamon

- 2 tbsp. of fresh lemon juice

Directions:

1. In a large pan, add water and apples on medium-low heat.

2. Simmer for about 10-15 minutes, stirring occasionally.

3. Remove from heat and keep aside to cool slightly.

4. In a blender, add apple mixture and pulse till smooth.

5. Return the mixture into pan on medium-low heat.

6. Stir in cinnamon and lemon juice and simmer for about 10 minutes.

7. Transfer the mixture onto dehydrator trays and with the back of spoon smooth the top.

8. Set the dehydrator at 135 degrees F.

9. Dehydrate for about 10-12 hours.

10. Cut the apple leather into equal sized rectangles.

11. Now, roll each rectangle to make fruit rolls.

Favorite Tea-Time Cookies (12 servings, serving: 1 portion)

Per Serving, Calories: 100- Fat: 1.1g - Carbs: 21.5g - Protein: 2.4g

Ingredients:

- ¼ cup of warm water

- 2 tsp. of chia seeds

- 2 cups of quick oats, divided

- ½ tsp. of baking soda

- ¾ tsp. of ground cinnamon

- ¼ tsp. of ground ginger

- ¼ tsp. of ground nutmeg

- ¼ cup of raisins

- 1 peeled, cored and chopped large apple

- 4 pitted and chopped Medjool dates

- 1 tsp. of apple cider vinegar

- 2 tbsp. of water

Directions:

1. Preheat the oven to 375 degrees F. Line a large cookie sheet with a large greased parchment paper.

2. In a bowl, mix together warm water and chia seeds. Keep aside till thickened.

3. In a large food processor, add 1 cup of of oats and pulse till grounded.

4. Transfer the ground oats in a large mixing bowl. Add remaining oats, baking soda, spices and raisins.

5. Now in blender, add remaining ingredients and pulse till smooth.

6. Transfer the apple mixture into the bowl with oat mixture and mix till well combined.

7. Stir in chia seeds mixture.

8. With a spoon, drop the mixture onto prepared cookie sheet. With your hands, flatten the cookies slightly.

9. Bake for about 12 minutes or till golden brown.

Delectable Scones (7 servings, serving: 1 portion)

Per Serving, Calories: 221- Fat: 17.6g - Carbs: 13.5g - Protein: 5.3g

Ingredients:

- 1 cup of almonds

- 1 1/3 cups of almond flour

- ¼ cup of arrowroot flour

- 1 tbsp. of coconut flour

- 1 tsp. of ground turmeric

- Pinch of sea salt

- Freshly ground black pepper, to taste

- 1 organic egg

- ¼ cup of olive oil

- 3 tbsp. of honey

- 1 tsp. of organic vanilla extract

Directions:

1. In a food processor, add almonds and pulse till chopped roughly

2. Transfer the chopped almonds in a large bowl.

3. Add flours and spices and mix well.

4. In another bowl, add remaining ingredients and beat till well combined.

5. Add flour mixture into egg mixture and mix till well combined.

6. Arrange a plastic wrap over cutting board.

7. Place the dough over cutting board.

8. With your hands, pat the dough into about 1-inch thick circle.

9. Carefully, cut the circle in 7 wedges.

10. Arrange the scones onto a cookie sheet in a single layer.

11. Bake for about 15-20 minutes.

Fiesta Savory Treat (8 servings, serving: 1 portion)

Per Serving, Calories: 139- Fat: 6.9g - Carbs: 13.6g - Protein: 7.1g

Ingredients:

- 2¼ cups of water

- ½ cup of green lentils

- 2 tsp. of olive oil

- 2 minced garlic cloves

- 2 cups of finely chopped cremini mushrooms

- 1 cup of finely chopped fresh spinach

- ½ tsp. of minced fresh thyme

- ½ tsp. of minced fresh rosemary

- 1/3 cup of finely chopped dried unsweetened cranberries

- ½ cup of toasted and finely chopped walnuts

- 1 tbsp. of fresh lemon juice

- 1 beaten organic egg

- ½ cup of roughly ground rolled oats

- Pinch of sea salt

- Pinch of crushed red pepper flakes

Directions:

1. Preheat your oven to 350 degrees F. Line a cookie sheet with a large parchment paper.

2. In a large pan, add water and lentil on high heat.

3. Reduce the heat to medium and simmer for about 20 minutes.

4. Remove from heat. With a potato masher, mash the lentils till a coarse paste forms. Keep aside.

5. Meanwhile in a large skillet, heat oil on medium-high heat.

6. Add garlic and sauté for about 1 minute.

7. Add mushrooms and cook for about 8 to 9 minutes.

8. Add spinach, herbs, cranberries, walnuts and lemon juice and cook for about 2 minutes.

9. Stir in mashed lentils and immediately remove from heat.

10. Keep aside to cool slightly.

11. Add oat flour and seasoning and mix till well combined.

12. Make desired size balls from mixture.

13. Arrange the balls onto prepared cookie sheet in a single layer.

14. Bake for about 15 minutes.

15. Gently, change the side of balls and bake for about 13 minutes more.

CHAPTER 5: DESSERT RECIPES

Elegant Stuffed Apples (4 servings, serving: 1 apple)

Per Serving, Calories: 204- Fat: 5.1g - Carbs: 42.1g - Protein: 2.5g

Ingredients:

- 4 peeled and cored large apples

- 2 tsp. of fresh lemon juice

- 1 cup of fresh blueberries

- ½ cup of fresh apple juice

- ½ tsp. of ground cinnamon

- ¼ cup of almond meal

- ¼ cup of unsweetened coconut flakes

Directions:

1. Preheat the oven to 375 degrees F.

2. Coat the apples with lemon juice evenly.

3. Arrange the apples in a baking dish.

4. Stuff each apple with blueberries.

5. Scatter the remaining blueberries around the apples and drizzle with apple juice.

6. Sprinkle each apple with cinnamon, almond meal and coconut flakes evenly.

7. Bake for about 30-35 minutes.

Summery Mango Delight (6 servings, serving: 1 portion)

Per Serving, Calories: 105- Fat: 0.1g - Carbs: 21.5g - Protein: 7g

Ingredients:

- 1½ cups of fat-free plain Greek yogurt

- 4½ cups of peeled, pitted and chopped frozen mango

- 2 drops of liquid stevia

Directions:

1. In a food processor, add all ingredients and pulse till smooth.

2. Serve immediately.

Creamy Ice-Cream (6 servings, serving: 1 portion)

Per Serving, Calories: 168- Fat: 10.3g - Carbs: 19.6g - Protein: 2.5g

Ingredients:

- 2 cups of pitted fresh cherries

- 1 peeled, pitted and chopped small avocado

- 10 pitted and chopped dates

- ¼ cup of soaked for 30 minutes and drained cashews

- 1¾ cups of unsweetened almond milk

- 2/3 cup of filtered water

- 1 tbsp. of fresh lemon juice

- 1 tbsp. of fresh beet juice

- 2 tbsp. of pitted and finely chopped fresh cherries

- ½ cup fresh whole cherries

Directions:

1. In a blender, add all ingredients except chopped and whole cherries and pulse till creamy and smooth.

2. Transfer into a bowl and stir in chopped cherries.

3. Now, transfer into an ice cream maker and process according to manufacturer's directions.

4. Transfer into an airtight container and freeze for at least 4-5 hours.

5. Top with fresh whole cherries and serve.

Refreshing Granita (8 servings, serving: 1 portion)

Per Serving, Calories: 85- Fat: 0.2g - Carbs: 22.2g - Protein: 0.6g

Ingredients:

- 1 cup of fresh blueberries

- 3 cups of sliced rhubarb

- ½ cup of honey

- 2½ cups of water

- 1 tbsp. of fresh mint leaves

Directions:

1. In a pan, add all ingredients on medium heat and cook for about 10 minutes, stirring occasionally.

2. Through a strainer, stain the mixture by pressing gently.

3. Discard the pulp of fruit.

4. Transfer the strained mixture into a 13x9-inch glass baking dish.

5. Freeze for about 20-30 minutes.

6. Remove from freezer and with a fork scrap the mixture.

7. Cover and freeze for about 1 hour, scraping after every 30 minutes.

Classic Pudding (3 servings, serving: 1 portion)

Per Serving, Calories: 370- Fat: 17.6g - Carbs: 50.4g - Protein: 10.2g

Ingredients:

- 1½ cups of peeled and roughly chopped carrot

- 6 tbsp. of chopped walnuts

- 3 tbsp. of honey

- 1 tsp. of ground cinnamon

- ¼ tsp. of ground ginger

- Pinch of ground nutmeg

- Pinch of ground cloves

- 2 cups of unsweetened almond milk

- 1 cup of water

- 1 tsp. of organic vanilla extract

- ¼ cup of chia seeds

Directions:

1. In a food processor, add carrot and walnuts and pulse until chopped finely.

2. Transfer the carrot mixture in a nonstick pan on medium heat.

3. Add honey and spices and cook for about 5-7 minutes, stirring occasionally.

4. Stir in almond milk, water and vanilla extract and remove from heat.

5. Transfer the mixture into a serving bowl.

6. Add chia seeds and stir to combine well.

7. Refrigerate, covered for overnight.

Family Favorite Pudding (4 servings, serving: 1 portion)

Per Serving, Calories: 243- Fat: 4.6g - Carbs: 12.5g - Protein: 39.7g

Ingredients:

- 1 cup of hulled and sliced fresh strawberries

- 1/3 cup of fresh blackberries

- 1/3 cup of fresh blueberries

- 12-ounce of drained silken tofu

- 2 scoops of unsweetened protein powder

- 1 tsp. of vanilla extract

- 1 tbsp. of honey

- 1 tsp. of pumpkin pie spice

Directions:

1. In a food processor, add all ingredients except raspberries and pulse till smooth.

2. Transfer into a serving glass and refrigerate for at least 2 hours before serving.

Traditional Holiday Pudding (4 servings, serving: 1 portion)

Per Serving, Calories: 169- Fat: 5.8g - Carbs: 31g - Protein: 1.6g

Ingredients:

- ¾ cup of homemade pumpkin puree

- 1 peeled and sliced ripe banana

- ½ of peeled, pitted and chopped avocado

- ¼ cup of honey

- ¼ cup of almond butter

- 1 tsp. of ground cinnamon

- ¼ tsp. of ground ginger

- ¼ tsp. of ground nutmeg

- ¼ tsp. of salt

- 1 tsp. of organic vanilla extract

Directions:

1. In a food processor, add all ingredients and pulse till smooth.

2. Divide pudding into 4 serving bowls.

3. Refrigerate for at least 2 hours before serving.

Sweet-Tooth Carving Custard (8 servings, serving: 1 portion)

Per Serving, Calories: 165- Fat: 13.4g - Carbs: 9.7g - Protein: 3.5g

Ingredients:

- 14-ounce of unsweetened coconut milk

- 2 peeled and finely mashed ripe bananas

- 3 organic eggs

- ½ tsp. of organic vanilla extract

Directions:

1. Preheat the oven to 350 degrees F. Lightly, grease 8 (6-inch) custard glasses. Arrange the glasses in a large baking dish.

2. In a large bowl, add all ingredients and mix till well combined.

3. Divide the banana mixture in prepared glasses evenly.

4. Pour water in the baking dish, about half way full.

5. Bake for about 20-25 minutes.

Thanksgiving Party Mousse (4 servings, serving: 1 portion)

Per Serving, Calories: 245- Fat: 14.3g - Carbs: 27.8g - Protein: 2g

Ingredients:

- 1 cup of unsweetened coconut milk

- 8-ounce of fresh cranberries

- ¼ cup of honey

- 3 tbsp. of fresh orange juice

- 1 tsp. of vanilla extract

- 1 tbsp. of vegan gelatin

- 2 tsp. of finely grated fresh orange zest

- 2 tbsp. of finely chopped fresh mint leaves

Directions:

1. In a high speed blender, add coconut milk and cranberries and pulse till smooth.

2. Add honey, orange juice and vanilla and pulse till well combined.

3. Through a fine sieve, strain the mixture into a pan on medium heat.

4. Heat the mixture for about 2 minutes and remove from heat.

5. Slowly, add gelatin, stirring continuously till dissolved completely.

6. Fold in orange zest and mint.

7. Transfer the mixture into 4 serving bowls

8. Refrigerate for about 1-4 hours or till set completely.

Luscious Cheesecake (8 servings, serving: 1 portion)

Per Serving, Calories: 106- Fat: 1.6g - Carbs: 19.6g - Protein: 5.1g

Ingredients:

- 2½ cups of low-fat Greek yogurt

- 6-8 drops of liquid stevia

- 3 organic egg whites

- 1/3 cup of raw cacao powder

- ¼ cup of arrowroot starch

- 1 tsp. of organic vanilla extract

- Pinch of sea salt

Directions:

1. Preheat the oven to 35 degrees F. Grease a 9-inch cake pan.

2. In a large bowl, add all ingredients and mix till well combined.

3. Place the mixture into prepared pan evenly.

4. Bake for about 30-35 minutes. Remove from oven and let it cool completely.

5. Refrigerate to chill for about 3-4 hours or till set completely.

6. Cut into 8 equal sized slices and serve.

Stunning Strawberry Sundae (2 servings, serving: 1 portion)

Per Serving, Calories: 122- Fat: 6g - Carbs: 7g - Protein: 7.8g

Ingredients:

- ½ cup of low-fat ricotta cheese

- 2 tsp. of organic vanilla extract

- 2 tsp. of fresh lemon juice

- 4 drops of liquid stevia

- ½ cup of hulled and sliced strawberries

- 2 tsp. of chopped almonds

Directions:

1. In a bowl, add all ingredients except strawberries and beat till smooth.

2. In a serving glass, place ¼ of cheese mixture and top with ½ of strawberries.

3. Top with ½ of remaining cheese mixture evenly.

4. Repeat with the remaining glass and mixture.

5. Serve immediately.

Celebratory Crisp (8 servings, serving: 1 portion)

Per Serving, Calories: 284- Fat: 21.4g - Carbs: 24.8g - Protein: 2.7g

Ingredients:

For Filling:

- 2 cups of peeled, cored and thinly sliced Granny Smith apples

- 1 cup of peeled, cored and thinly sliced Fuji apple

- 1 cup of fresh cranberries

- Pinch of ground nutmeg

- Pinch of ground cinnamon

- 1 tbsp. of fresh lemon juice

For Topping:

- ¼ cup of finely chopped pecans

- 1 cup of almond flour

- ¼ cup of pitted and finely chopped dates

- ½ tsp. of ground cinnamon

- Pinch of sea salt

- 3 tbsp. of maple syrup

- 1/3 cup of extra-virgin olive oil

Directions:

1. Preheat the oven to 375 degrees F. Grease a 9x9-inch baking dish.

2. In a large bowl, add all filling ingredients and toss to coat well.

3. Transfer the fruit mixture in the bottom of prepared baking dish evenly.

4. For topping in the same bowl, add all filling ingredients and toss to coat well.

5. Spread the topping mixture over filling evenly.

6. Bake for about 40 minutes or till top becomes golden brown.

Exotic Crumble (4 servings, serving: 1 portion)

Per Serving, Calories: 206- Fat: 13.6g - Carbs: 17.3g - Protein: 7.1g

Ingredients:

For Filling:

- 1½ cups of hulled and chopped fresh strawberries

- 1 tsp. of arrowroot starch

For Topping:

- ½ cup of oat flour

- 2 tbsp. of almond flour

- 1½ tbsp. of almond butter

- 2 tbsp. of chopped walnuts

- ¼ tsp. of ground cinnamon

Directions:

1. Preheat the oven to 350 degrees F. Lightly, grease a baking dish.

2. Place strawberries in the bottom of prepared baking dish.

3. Sprinkle with arrowroot starch and gently stir to combine.

4. In a bowl, mix together all topping ingredients.

5. Spread the topping mixture over strawberries evenly.

6. Bake for about 20-25 minutes or till top becomes golden brown.

Kid's Favorite Mini Cakes (6 servings, serving: 1 mini cake)

Per Serving, Calories: 201- Fat: 12.8g - Carbs: 20.6g - Protein: 3.5g

Ingredients:

- ¾ cup of pitted and chopped fresh cherries

- ¼ teaspoon vanilla bean powder, divided

- 1/3 cup of honey, divided

- 1¼ cups of almond flour

- ¼ tsp. of baking soda

- Pinch of sea salt

- ¼ cup of extra-virgin olive oil

- 2 organic eggs

- 1 tsp. of organic vanilla extract

Directions:

1. Preheat the oven to 350 degrees F. Grease 6 cups of a muffin tray.

2. In a bowl, mix together cherries, 1/8 teaspoon of vanilla bean powder and 2 tablespoons of honey.

3. In a second bowl, mix together flour, baking soda and salt.

4. In a third bowl, add oil, eggs, almond extract and remaining honey and vanilla bean powder and beat till well combined.

5. Add flour mixture into egg mixture and mix till well combined.

6. Place the cherry mixture into prepared muffin cups evenly.

7. Top with flour mixture evenly.

8. Bake for about 20 minutes.

9. Carefully invert the cakes onto serving plates.

Quickest Zesty Cake (1 serving, serving: 1 cake)

Per Serving, Calories: 337- Fat: 14.7g - Carbs: 45.6g - Protein: 10.8g

Ingredients:

- 1½ tbsp. of coconut flour

- ½ tbsp. of baking powder

- Pinch of sea salt

- 1 organic egg

- 1 tbsp. of unsweetened coconut milk

- 2 tbsp. of fresh lime juice

- 1 tsp. of finely grated fresh lime zest

- 1 peeled and mashed banana

- 2 tbsp. of shredded unsweetened coconut

Directions:

1. Lightly, grease a microwave safe mug.

2. In a bowl, mix together flour, baking powder and salt.

3. In another bowl, add egg, coconut milk, lime juice, lime zest and banana and beat till well combined.

4. Add flour mixture into banana mixture and mix till well combined.

5. Fold in coconut.

6. Transfer the mixture into prepared mug.

7. Microwave on High for about 2-2½ minutes.

8. Remove from microwave and keep aside to cool before serving.

Final Words

Thank you again for picking up this cookbook! I hope it was able to help you to find a wide variety of simple, and delicious sounding recipes that you can't wait to try for yourself.

Finally, if you enjoyed this book, then I'd like to ask you for a favor, would you be kind enough to leave a review for this book? It'd be greatly appreciated!